Put Insomnia to Sleep

Retrain your brain for an amazing sleep

Helen Dugdale

First published by Ultimate World Publishing 2023

ISBN

Paperback: 978-1-922982-48-3
Ebook: 978-1-922982-49-0

Cover design: Ultimate World Publishing
Layout and typesetting: Ultimate World Publishing
Editor: Vanessa McKay

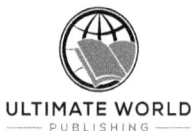

Ultimate World Publishing
Diamond Creek,
Victoria Australia 3089
www.writeabook.com.au

Foreword

W/hen I received my copy of Helen Dugdale's new book, Put Insomnia to Sleep, I knew that what I was about to read will be typically Helen. Those of us that have the good fortune to know Helen will know she is one of the most interesting people we have met.

Helen Dugdale has two defining strengths that I was confident would set this book above the noise of the competitive conversation in the health and well-being sector.

Firstly, Helen is erudite. The information she has provided in the book is the result of scholarly research and innate wisdom. She has referenced the science and distilled the research to form and understand the complex thesis that sleep, with diet and exercise, is the magic link to physical health and mental well-being.

As I read the book, I began to understand that sleep is the missing link in our well-being. Sleep is the aspect of our health to which we pay the least attention, has the most impact and is in our control. I kept coming back to the quote that Helen has used from Thomas Decker, "Sleep is the golden chain that holds the body and soul together". It became apparent to me that sleep is more than physical health, it is the key to our emotional and mental well-being.

Helen's research and insight into the challenge of putting insomnia to sleep has created this important book.

Secondly, Helen gives of herself with unbridled generosity. My own experience is that Helen cares deeply about the people she assists. I have seen her involved in many community programs, activities and events that demonstrate and display her selflessness. In the work that I have been involved with Helen over many years, it is her level of care that is not just obvious, but outstanding.

The Brain Coaching work she has been doing over a long period is based on care. I am one of many that have been carefully guided through the Brain Coaching process to address my own sleep problem. Helen helped me identify a problem that I was not even aware of. She found in me a roadblock that was deeper in me than I had allowed myself to venture. We had a cathartic revelation that thoroughly surprised me.

The revelation then led to tools and a process to resolve my circumstance and retrain my mind to leave it behind. Helen taught me to move on from my roadblock.

I slept. I learnt to sleep with the assurance that I had resolved my inner anxiety.

I do hope you enjoy this book and getting to know Helen Dugdale as much as I have.

Mike Logan AM

Dedication

To my three wonderful grandchildren –
Angus, Connor and Amelia.
"You can do anything, be anything you want,
if you set your mind to it."

Contents

Introduction

"Sleep – we all do it, but only about half of us do it well!"
(Unknown author)

This was an interesting quote I saw a few years ago by an anonymous person.

I thought, that would be funny if it wasn't so true. Research shows that about 40-50% of the population in most Western countries has one or more sleep problems[1.]

While so many people suffer from sleep problems, many of my Brain Coaching clients are successfully overcoming their insomnia. Before I delve into how to overcome insomnia, let me answer a question many people ask me: what made me become a Brain Coach?

After decades of teaching and working in research and development, I started my own personal development business – facilitating workshops to help people get the best out of themselves and the people around them. I then went back to university in 2014 and studied Psychology, to learn more about how our brains work, and to further help others. After I enrolled in the Post Graduate Diploma of Psychology at the University of New England, I was talking to my good friend in Germany about what I was doing, and she said that she was studying psychology as well. She told me about an excellent program developed by German psychologists about ten years earlier. I did my research and went to Europe in October 2014 to train in this method. Since then, I have helped over 500 people Australia-wide, as well as international clients, with their anxieties, fears, phobias, and performance.

Then Covid hit in early 2020 and I couldn't see as many clients face-to-face. This gave me plenty of time to think and I decided to write a book! I thought of all the clients I meet with sleeping problems. Addressing their sleep issues, in turn, reduced their stress and resolved all sorts of other issues. In late 2020, I started researching and writing this book to share my Brain Coaching method. I wanted to let more people know that practical help is available, that it is not expensive, nor intrusive, and does not require pharmaceuticals.

Another reason I chose the topic of insomnia was because I suffered insomnia for a long time, and I know exactly what people are going through when they can't sleep. I even ran the London marathon on only five hours of sleep. You *can* perform on little sleep if you persevere, but I wouldn't recommend this as a long-term strategy! I know people who have stayed up all night studying for exams or to finish a project. You *can* do it. You can perform the next day, but not every day. Sleep deprivation will take its toll.

Clients tell me they've tried everything and nothing works, then they stress further about whether they will sleep. I understand. I relate to people who are suffering from insomnia and all the daily consequences that follow. I have tried most of the so-called 'remedies' available and have had marginal success with some of them. In the back of this book, I have listed the top tips that have helped me and my clients. *They work!* Believe me, it is amazing to wake up feeling refreshed and raring to go for the day without the need for pharmaceuticals. You really have to give each strategy time to see if they will work for you, time for each to become a habit. That is what brain re-training is all about. And you are never too old to start new habits. As Aristotle said about 2300 years ago – *"we are what we repeatedly do"*.

In this book, you will find the science behind why sleep is so important. You don't have to put up with sleepless nights and the consequences. I outline the benefits of good sleep, share plenty of handy tips, with guidelines on how to improve your sleeping environment, your medical and physical issues. I also introduce how Brain Coaching improves your emotional well-being in order to get a good sleep.

On my journey as a Brain Coach, researching insomnia and helping people to overcome sleep problems, I have developed a sleep workshop program, a sleep quiz, and a comprehensive sleep diary. Word-of-mouth and social media sharing have guided many clients to me for help when they haven't been able to find relief elsewhere. They have told me they feel amazing after working with me, and that my sleep program has improved their lives and relationships.

By taking advantage of our brain's plasticity, it is possible to change old habits and thought patterns and create new positive pathways of thinking. Regardless of age, we can rewire our brains and form new healthy habits.

Whatever the reason for your insomnia, Brain Coaching can help you. Close your eyes and imagine how energised and clear-headed you will feel after refreshing nights of good sleep. You will be more productive, healthier, and may even live longer.

CHAPTER 1

Importance of Sleep

"Lack of sleep is only bad if you have to drive, think, talk or move."
Dov Davidoff.

Sleep is essential for life. We feel and look better when we get a good night's sleep. While we sleep, our body regenerates cells and tissue, repairs damage to muscles, nerves and organs, and boosts our immune system. During sleep, our brain refines and repairs thought pathways, processes, resolves emotional events, and stores new memories. Have you ever gone to bed stewing over something and, after a good night's sleep, the problem doesn't seem as bad as you thought?

When we don't get a good night's sleep, issues or worries may seem worse the next day. We feel more emotional, our responses and reactions are impaired, and life is just harder. There are many reasons for interruptions to our sleep. When sleep interruptions persist, we graduate from occasional sleeplessness into insomnia.

Insomnia: "difficulty in initiating or maintaining a restorative sleep, which results in fatigue, the severity or persistence of which causes clinically significant distress or impairment in functioning. Such sleeplessness may be caused by a transient or chronic physical condition or psychological disturbance."[1] American Psychological Association

When we don't get enough sleep, we feel constantly tired and emotional, and can spend our life walking around like we have a hangover. We don't function as well at work and our relationships suffer. We experience a downward spiral in our quality of life. We take substances like alcohol, drugs, pharmaceuticals or supplements. We try other sorts of remedies like lavender pillows, running around the block, and the list goes on. How many activities or remedies have you tried?

The dangers of not sleeping well have been cited in relation to many serious accidents, including the Chernobyl Nuclear Disaster, plane and train crashes, even the Challenger Space Shuttle crash[2]. Tiredness is often a contributing factor in many everyday major and minor accidents at workplaces or on the road. Have you ever noticed the signs on country roads warning of driver fatigue? Tiredness can be as dangerous as drink-driving.

A significant danger of poor sleep is the temptation to take more and more sleeping pills. Some people are so desperate for sleep that they'll consider, 'If two tablets worked for a while, but I *still* can't sleep, then I'll try four tablets,' and so on. In some instances, the longer we use a drug, the more our body needs to achieve the same effect. Some people are so desperate for sleep that they ignore the label warnings by taking more tablets to get some sleep. They may accidentally over-dose, not on purpose, but out of desperation.

Being sleep-deprived affects our judgement. We can't think rationally when all we want to do is sleep. Sadly, you may be aware of celebrities or people in the public eye who have accidentally overdosed on sleeping pills. These fatalities have helped raise the awareness of accidental overdose and sleeping issues. As a Brain Coach, I know this situation can be avoided. Please speak to your doctor or pharmacist if you are taking sleeping tablets. There are warnings on the label about the length of time you should take them and how their effectiveness can wear off with continued use.

I have clients who experience increased anxiety about being unable to sleep. Each night, they stress about the upcoming night ahead, and if they will get enough sleep. This worry adds to their stress, making it even less likely for them to get a good night's sleep. The more worry they have around the amount of sleep, the less sleep they have. The less sleep they have, the more they stress and worry. For many, this exhausting routine will continue to disrupt life until the cycle is broken.

Good quality sleep includes the REM stage (Rapid Eye Movement) where the left and right hemispheres of the brain resolve the day's emotional issues. If you've ever gone to bed worrying over something, and woken up the following day thinking, *'It's not that bad. What was I worried about?'* REM has done its job! Of course, a good night's sleep won't solve major dramas in your life, but it can help you deal with them more effectively.

When we don't get enough sleep, our immune system becomes compromised. Have you ever noticed that you are more likely to get sick when you are tired and feel run down? Your resistance to sore throats, headaches, stomach problems, aches, and pain is lowered. Ongoing sleep deprivation can negatively affect your immune system and reduce your body's ability to respond to infections and other diseases.

Sleep deprivation can affect our food choices. Sleep-deprived people tend to eat more of the unhealthy stuff – usually sugar, caffeine or fat to boost their energy and concentration. They justify it by saying, '*I'll just have a chocolate bar to get me through the afternoon.*' When feeling tired and bothered, it can just be too much effort to prepare healthy snacks or meals.

Sleep deprivation can increase the risk of obesity, and obesity can lead to breathing problems inhibiting quality sleep. It is not unusual for people to gain weight, not only because of poor food choices, but because a lack of sleep keeps us in a state of heightened stress. The stress hormone, cortisol, increases the release of glucose into our system, readying us for the fight-or-flight reaction, but without an actual physical threat to use up that extra energy, it gets stored as fat[3]. When daily stress persists to bedtime, it can cause us to fight sleep, disrupting our circadian rhythm (our body clock), affecting the production of calming sleep hormones. A lack of sleep can adversely affect the production of hormones needed for proper body function, indirectly leading to weight gain.

Have you felt so tired that you don't feel like exercising? We know that physical activity is good for fitness, mental well-being, circulation, and supplying oxygen to blood and brain cells. Feeling too tired to move gives us another reason to feel bad about ourselves for not keeping up a healthy routine. It's hard to sit back and watch our mental and physical health decline. Pushing through and getting in some form of movement, even a short walk, helps our well-being.

Sleep is critical for our physical health. Healing and repair take place while we sleep. During sleep, our heart rate, breathing, and blood pressure reduce and this is thought to enhance conditions for circulation and organ repair. Continued sleep problems can lead to an increased risk of heart disease, kidney disease, high blood pressure, diabetes, and stroke, amongst many other health conditions[4].

Yes, 'beauty sleep' is a thing! A lack of sleep not only affects our mental and physical health, but it also affects our physical appearance. People notice we look tired when we haven't had enough sleep. Why does our face sag and look sallow, and why do bags develop under our eyes when we have interrupted sleep, particularly for days on end? It all stems back to the physiology of cell regeneration and repair that occurs when we sleep. (As skin is the body's largest organ, there is a lot of cell regeneration). A research trial in 2013 by Sundelin et al., identified the following noticeable signs after participants had only a few nights of poor sleep: hanging eyelids; swollen eyes; dark circles under eyes; paler skin; more wrinkles and fine lines; droopy corners of the mouth[5]. Dark circles under the eyes are caused by blood vessels dilating. The dilation is most noticeable under the eyes because the skin here is thinner. During a good sleep, blood flow increases to the skin, helping to rehydrate skin cells, build collagen, repair cell damage, and reduce the onset of wrinkles.

When you sleep, melatonin production increases. Melatonin acts as an antioxidant and helps minimise the ageing effect. When cortisol (stress hormone) levels decrease during sleep, skin repair is improved. As you sleep, collagen production increases, helping minimise fine lines. During sleep, the production of human growth hormone increases, strengthening skin. Excess cortisol levels, because of a lack of sleep, can lead to an increase in sebum, the secretion from the sebaceous glands. Too much sebum can lead to oily skin and inflammation of skin rashes including eczema, psoriasis, and dermatitis. Too little sebum can lead to dry, itchy skin. A study by Oyetakin-White et al. found that - "*chronic poor sleep quality is associated with increased signs of intrinsic ageing, diminished skin barrier function and lower satisfaction with appearance*"[6].

Poor sleep causes the skin to age faster[6], and inhibits recovery from exposure to the environment, such as wind, sun and dry air. When you wake up feeling and looking tired, not only is your mood affected, but how you look can inadvertently worry others. Friends, family or colleagues might presume that you are sad, depressed or angry, and react to you differently. Are you tired of looking tired?

Good quality sleep supports growth and development, which is why it is so vital for children and teenagers to get adequate sleep. Sleep is essential for everyone: to rid the body of toxins (possibly reducing the chance of Alzheimer's), helping to lay down new memories, reducing anxiety, and regulating moods. Adequate sleep is also good therapy for other ailments. The body can fight infections while sleeping. The brain can resolve emotional issues while sleeping, especially during REM sleep, helping to reduce susceptibility to anxiety and depression.

CASE STUDIES

Sean is in his late 40's and has only ever had 2 hours sleep a night for the past 20 years. He told me that some nights he didn't sleep at all! I asked, "How do you get through the day?", and his reply was, "Only just". After 3 sessions of Brain Coaching, he regularly sleeps 8 hours per night. Now Sean says, "I can't believe how much energy I have!". His daily routine is to make healthy eating choices, with no caffeine after midday. Sean also meditates and sometimes does some gentle stretches. He might have a glass of wine with dinner, then a warm shower prior to bedtime, he then repeats a positive mantra, listens to binaural beats music and reads a book before he turns the lights out.

Sean sleeps from about 10.30pm to 6.30am and wakes up refreshed and ready for a productive day. He is happy and calm, looks forward to being sociable, and loves being with people. "Since I am sleeping better, there are so many positive 'flow-on' impacts in the rest of my life".

Steve is a new client, in his 50's - he is not very happy with himself, and he does not enjoy being with people in his current state of mind. He only sleeps about 4 hours per night, makes unhealthy food choices because he is so tired, he doesn't care and 'can't be bothered' to do anything nice for himself. Steve puts off going to bed and is on social media until about 2am, even though he needs to get up at about 6.30. Because he is on his screen till the early hours, his brain is stimulated, cortisol and adrenalin are racing around in his system, his body clock is out of sync, and it is hard for him to go to sleep. He said that he is tired and grumpy, and nobody wants to be with him when he is like that, and he doesn't want to be with anyone either. He said he just 'wants to lock himself away'. He doesn't want to do anything, lacks motivation big time, has given up doing any exercises (which he used to really enjoy). Because Steve is tired all the time, not exercising and making unhealthy food choices, his health is suffering in other areas, too. Everything seems to be snowballing and poor Steve feels that he is in a vicious cycle of poor sleep, poor everything. The people around him seem to be getting annoyed with him, too. *How on earth is he is going to get out of this cycle?*

Brain Coaching can help him prioritise what he really wants to do, encourage him to introduce better personal habits, and have better quality sleep.

Chapter summary

Sleep is essential for our physical, mental, and emotional health. A lack of sleep not only affects the individual, but impacts our family and relationships, our workplace, and society as a whole. Sleeping well not only relieves stress and anxiety, but increases alertness, memory, and productivity. Sleep improves immunity against infections and diseases. It can be a relatively inexpensive form of therapy for many ailments, reducing an unnecessary drain on the health system. Adequate sleep can help to reduce the number of accidents, decrease reliance on pharmaceuticals, and reduce the incidence of mental disorders.

There are many reasons to improve our sleep. So why do we continue to put up with sleep problems? In my practice, I hear comments like:

- I've always been like this.
- I've tried everything.
- I've learnt to cope.
- It's just how my brain is wired.
- I'm so tired, it's all I can do to get through the day.
- I don't know how to change.

Some people are even proud of how they can get by on so little sleep! We all know something has to give if sleepless nights continue – their health, their relationships, or their work will suffer. Some say that they can't afford treatment, or that nothing they've tried works. They lack motivation and energy, or they may have become depressed or despondent and feel that there is no hope for improvement.

To improve your sleeping patterns, you need to investigate whether you have a medical problem. If so, medical advice should be followed as the first step in recovering a healthy sleep routine. Brain Coaching can help motivate you to follow through with changes recommended by your medical practitioner.

You might discover an environmental problem is disturbing your sleep – noise, or bright lights, for example. In many instances, environmental disturbances are easy and quick to remediate.

There could be a physiological problem rather than a medical one, and a simple 'body hack' could help improve your sleep issue. You could try avoiding caffeine at night or change the timing of your exercise. Brain Coaching will help identify issues, create and reinforce new strategies, and help you set up your new daily routine in order to get a good night's sleep.

Suppose you have sorted through the possible environmental, medical, and physiological reasons preventing you from achieving good quality sleep. You may need to look into the possibility of emotional reasons for your chronic insomnia. Your logical mind knows all the reasons you need a good night's sleep, so let's find out what is stopping you.

CASE STUDY

Tom lives in a capital city. He is anxious about many parts of his life, for example: driving in traffic, being alone on back roads, and he worries about his adult son. Tom is anxious about so many things that sometimes he can't eat, so you can imagine his concentration at work is low. He can't sleep, can't eat, and suffers constant anxiety. He wakes up at about 3 am each morning and starts worrying about everything, especially about his son. So much so that his son was getting annoyed about the hovering and the interference in his life from his father, who loves him. Then Tom would start worrying about his relationship with his son, and how he was pushing him away with anxious behaviour. During the Brain Coaching session, we uncovered the original reason for his anxiety. He finally dealt with those buried feelings, introduced positive strategies to bring logical thinking into his daily dealings, and developed a nightly sleep routine. After putting his strategies in place, if he woke up, he could put himself back to sleep in no time. Waking up refreshed every day also meant he could think more logically about his driving anxiety, other behaviours, and the treatment of his son. They now have a much better, and more mutually respectful relationship. And as Tom said,

"I didn't even come to you about my sleeping problems, I came to you about my driving anxiety!" and he was laughing!

CHAPTER 2

Science of Sleep

"Sleep is the golden chain that ties body and soul together,"
Thomas Decker.

There are many processes at work within the body and brain during sleep. These interactive processes are directly linked to sleep satisfaction. Research is still being conducted on how and why all these processes interact. Complex processes, involving neurons in the brain and their signalling system connected to the rest of the body, stimulate the production of hormones and chemicals that affect sleep. Some of these processes are influenced by genes (epigenetics, passed down through generations) and some are impacted by environmental and lifestyle choices.

Why can't we function without sleep?

People who can get away with little sleep think that just resting is enough, that they don't actually need to sleep for long periods. Scientific studies are working towards determining why regular, deep sleep is so important for regenerative processes to take place. While we are just resting, rather than sleeping, our brains are still active - still thinking and processing. The functions the body carries out typically during sleep cannot happen as effectively when we are awake. Many systems in the body require quality sleep time in order to function properly. Sleep is vital for the proper functioning and maintenance of our:

- respiratory system
- digestive system
- cardiovascular system
- nervous system
- muscular system
- integumentary (skin) system
- skeletal system
- reproductive system
- endocrine (hormones) system
- immune system

When we don't get enough sleep, we put ourselves at risk for numerous health disorders: heart disease, digestive issues, diabetes, obesity, depression, and high blood pressure[1].

Let's dive a little deeper into some of the miraculous ways the science of sleep takes care of our bodies and minds. You've probably heard of the circadian rhythm. It's top on the list of sleep influencers.

Sleep and Circadian Rhythm

Circadian rhythm: *The natural cycle of physical, mental, and behaviour changes that the body goes through in a 24-hour cycle. Circadian rhythms are mostly affected by light and darkness and are controlled by a small area in the middle of the brain. They can affect sleep, body temperature, hormones, appetite, and other body functions. Abnormal circadian rhythms may be linked to obesity, diabetes, depression, bipolar disorder, seasonal affective disorder, and sleep disorders such as insomnia. Circadian rhythm is sometimes called the 'body's clock.'* National Institute of General Medical Science. (https://nigms.nih.gov/education/fact-sheets/Pages/circadian-rhythms.aspx)

Good sleep requires both quality sleep and quantity of sleep. Most adults need to sleep 7-8 hours a night to function properly the next day. Quality of sleep is measured by the depth of sleep, enabling the resolution of emotional issues, laying down of new memories, and removal of waste from the brain.

Our sleep cycle has four stages: Rapid Eye Movement (REM) sleep and three non-REM sleep stages. Each stage cycles us through specific brain wavelengths. We move through these four stages in around 90 minutes, a few times per night.

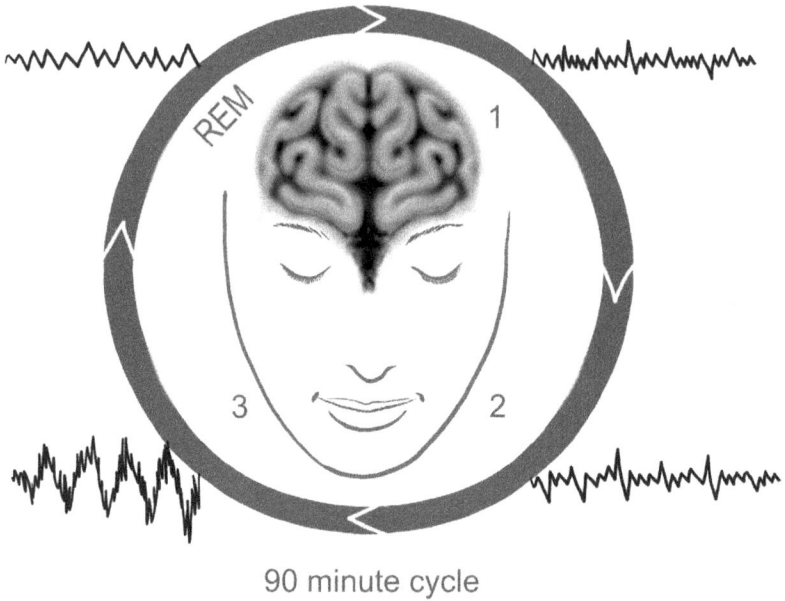

90 minute cycle

Diagram – Four Stages of Sleep
Original artwork: Graeme Compton

Non-REM sleep happens over three stages:

Stage 1 is the changeover from being awake to falling into a light sleep. Everything in your body winds down, including heart rate, breathing, and brain waves. Your muscles relax.

Stage 2 is still relatively light sleep before you enter deep sleep. Everything relaxes further - your body temperature drops, and your eye movements become still. If you do not have insomnia, most sleep is spent in this stage.

Stage 3 is a deep sleep. This is when restorative sleep occurs. Everything relaxes completely. Brainwaves have slowed even further. This stage of the cycle usually lasts longer in the earlier part of the night. It may be hard to wake up from a deep sleep because your muscles and brain are so relaxed.

Rapid Eye Movement (REM) sleep is the stage of sleep where your eyes flicker left and right, behind closed eyelids. The heart rate is almost the same as when awake, and breathing becomes faster. It is also called the paradoxical sleep - you are asleep, but not asleep. REM can occur a few times a night as you move through your cycles of sleep.

We know that during REM sleep, memories are consolidated, emotions are processed, and anxieties are resolved (to a certain degree). Achieving REM sleep enhances our ability to learn and leaves us feeling emotionally stable. This stage is also when vivid dreams occur due to increased brain activity.

A 2013 review[2], found that alcohol has a detrimental effect on the amount of REM sleep that occurs, decreasing memory and emotional stability. Many of us believe that alcohol can actually be a sleep aid but research shows the opposite is true. While the effects of alcohol are initially relaxing, even numbing, the physiology shows that using alcohol to induce sleep can be detrimental in the long term. Not only can you wake up with a hangover, but you suffer the loss of beneficial REM sleep.

Rick Wassing et al. (2016), in their study of REM[3], found that emotions are destabilised, memories are disrupted, and anxiety can build up when REM is disrupted. Disrupted REM sleep can lead to a cycle of insomnia – you feel anxious, your sleep is disturbed, then because you haven't had enough sleep, you become more anxious. Before you realise, insomnia has become a habit, and you are left more emotionally vulnerable.

Sleep and Brain Detoxification

Waste materials are removed from the brain while we sleep. The glymphatic drainage system removes the daily build-up of toxic waste in and around the brain during sleep. Neurobiologist Moheb Costandi (2018) described the glymphatic drainage system as a waste disposal system for the brain. *"It consists of a network of vessels that run alongside blood vessels in the brain and drains waste-filled cerebrospinal fluid (CSF) from the brain."*[4] If this doesn't happen, because we haven't had enough good quality sleep, a plaque of toxins and proteins can build up around brain cells, and scientists believe that this is how Alzheimer's begins. (Note: Not all insomniacs get Alzheimer's, but lack of sleep can be a warning sign). Think of this system like a busy city, where it is more efficient to collect the garbage during the night, when the roads are less busy, and the garbage removal is less likely to be interrupted by traffic. The brain cannot process sensory information like sight, sound, taste, and clear away waste simultaneously. Our brain must wait until sleep takes over and there is no sensory activity. Prolonged periods of insomnia will mean these waste products may accumulate to toxic levels and could impair sleep even further[5].

Sleep and the Heart

Regular sleep is important for a healthy cardiovascular system. Interrupted or insufficient sleep can lead to problems with blood pressure, and increase the risk of heart disease, heart attacks or stroke. Our heart rate normally slows down during normal, sufficient non-REM sleep stages, and blood pressure drops by about 10-20%, reducing heart stress. When a person doesn't get enough deep sleep, blood pressure may not decrease, leading to hypertension and the risk of stroke. Poor sleep has also been known to trigger chronic inflammation, implicated in the build-up of plaque lining the arteries, leading to hardening of the arteries. Hypertension can strain the arteries, making them less efficient at bringing blood to the heart. One study found that poor sleep increased the chance of heart attack by 20%[6]. Non-REM sleep helps the heart slow down; and during REM stage sleep, the heart rate speeds up. When these stages of sleep are not completed, the risk of adverse heart conditions could arise.

Sleep and the Liver

Insufficient or interrupted sleep can contribute to fatty liver disease[7]. The liver's function is to break down fat cells; if this is compromised, disease can result. Other factors also contribute to fatty liver disease, but if we can improve our sleep, we deal with one less risk factor. The liver is synchronised with our circadian rhythm, linking the sleep/wake and detoxification cycles. The liver is also involved in regulating hormones, nutrient metabolism, detoxifying the body, and processing insulin. If sleep is insufficient, then all the above functions will be compromised.

Sleep and the Lungs

Insufficient sleep can reduce lung function, and compromised lung function can impact sleep[8]. Sleep influences mucus retention, bronchial reactions, and respiration, especially during REM sleep stage, when breathing is more shallow and less frequent. Breathing difficulties of any kind can affect lung function.

Sleep and Metabolism

Recent research suggests that in addition to diet and exercise, sleep impacts our metabolism (how the body converts food to energy). During normal sleep, our metabolic rate drops by around 15% and is at its lowest in the mornings. This doesn't sound like much of a reduction, but metabolising at this level is optimal. Reduced sleep can encourage weight gain and the risk of diabetes. Other studies have found that even a week of insufficient sleep can cause a significant alteration in metabolic and endocrine (hormone) levels.[9]

Sleep and Immune Function

The immune system is fundamental for the health of our body – it heals wounds, fights infections, and helps protect against chronic diseases. As with other systems in our body, sleep and our immune system have a bidirectional effect. For example – a viral infection can impact our sleep; disrupted sleep can decrease our ability to fight off infections. *"During sleep, your immune system releases proteins called cytokines, some of which help promote sleep. Certain cytokines need to increase when you have an infection or inflammation, or when you're under stress. Sleep deprivation may decrease production of these protective cytokines."* Dr. Eric Olson, Mayo Clinic.

Scientists have found that certain functions of the immune system are activated during sleep and help fight inflammation. They also found that sleep helps the immune system to 'remember' or to recognise dangerous antigens in our system. Scientists believe that this occurs because our breathing and muscle activity have slowed during sleep, thus conserving energy which is used to fight inflammation. When we aren't sleeping, we aren't conserving this energy to fight off infections. Scientists also believe that melatonin, a hormone mainly prevalent during nighttime hours, is involved in this process. Many studies show that statistically, people who continually get less than 6 hours sleep tend to get sick more often, have more colds and flus, and are at greater risk of developing other diseases. Insufficient sleep seems to interfere with healthy immune function and inflammation persists. Sometimes, an infection can alter how much time is spent in certain sleep stages. Therefore, sometimes when we are sick, we spend more time in deep sleep, which aids our immune response. Deep sleep involves the slowing down of bodily processes, allowing the immune system to utilise more energy to fight infection.[10]

Sleep and Mood

There is a bidirectional link between quality of sleep and regulation of emotions and mood. Insufficient sleep makes people more emotionally aroused or upset. They have more sensitive reactions to events and stimuli than people who sleep well. The opposite follows, where adverse emotional responses to daily activities can lead to sleep disturbances. Research has shown that when people can adapt to stressful situations and put in place strategies that help them sleep better, they are likely to be more emotionally stable. It comes down to the amount of non-REM sleep and REM sleep that a person can experience each night. Insomniacs report that they have more trouble coping with daily stressors than people who sleep well.

Sleeping problems may be both a cause of, and a result of emotional problems.

Worry, anxiety and fear can bring a person to a state of 'hyperarousal' that is difficult to overcome or calm down from. As a result, it can become difficult to get to sleep or get back to sleep. If a person is not getting enough quality sleep, especially in the REM stage where emotions are regulated, then this hyper state can continue into the daytime, adversely affecting their mood.

Sufficient good quality sleep is essential for general well-being, considering that non-REM sleep and REM sleep play a regulating role on our emotions experienced during the day. Sleep deprivation can predetermine disorders like depression. *"Healthy sleep repairs adaptive processing, functional brain activity, integrity of the connections between the medial prefrontal cortex and the amygdala, and thus improves the capacity to regulate emotions as well as an individual's well-being."*[11.] (Vandekerckhove)

Chapter Summary

When we take the time to investigate some of the science behind the purpose of sleep, we find that a healthy regular sleep routine is vital for the proper functioning of a vibrant body and mind. Implementing a regular, calming sleep routine needs to be our top priority. This puts us in a good frame of mind and lets our body know to relax and wind down for the day. Our circadian rhythm does its job, melatonin kicks in, cortisol goes down, the feel-good hormones go up, and our heart rate and blood pressure start slowing down.

Sleep is a wonderful, inexpensive therapy for many disorders.

Getting a good night's sleep helps to maintain health and avoid a physical and/or mental decline. Good quality sleep keeps us more emotionally stable, enhances memory function, enables us to fight infections effectively, helps our organs function better, and keeps our skin looking great! If you are suffering from insomnia or other sleep disorders, you may already be experiencing a follow-on effect of health issues. Note that not all insomniacs will have major health issues, it's just that continuous poor sleep increases your chances of something going wrong. It's a bit like smoking, - not all smokers get lung cancer – but we know the dangers of smoking.

> *"Sleep is the best cognitive enhancer we have to target psychological, neurological, and physiological disorders."* Russell Foster (Uni Oxford, 2013).

CHAPTER 3

Breaking Bad
Sleeping Habits

"Me: Let me Sleep;
Brain: LOL no, let's stay awake and
remember all the stupid things you've ever done.
Me: okay".

Bad habits are hard to break, for example:

- chewing your nails,
- saying 'but' after everything,
- interrupting people,
- cracking your knuckles,
- playing on your phone till all hours of the night and then being unable to sleep.

People do these things without thinking. That's what a habit is.

We can change our behaviour so that good habits are what we do without thinking.

Habits to Avoid

Poor habits before bedtime can lead to poor sleep because certain bad habits stimulate the brain and raise the levels of stress hormones, cortisol, and adrenalin. Once our bodies and brain have established poor sleeping habits, the habits become a persistent pattern. Our bodies become used to waking up after a few hours and not being able to get back to sleep, or taking longer to get to sleep. Poor sleep habits set up a relentless cycle of insufficient sleep.

Here are some habits to avoid, especially prior to sleep:

- **Coffee** in the late afternoon or evenings: can stimulate you for up to 10 hours while caffeine is in your system, keeping you alert.
- **Big meals**, especially later at night, can lead to a heaviness in the stomach and your system working hard to digest food, keeping your system active rather than winding down.
- **Alcohol** late in the evening: can initially put you to sleep but may wake you later as your liver works to metabolise the alcohol; it also could lead to the need to urinate during the night and cause headaches from dehydration.
- **Exercise** workouts at night: can lead to adrenalin being pumped around the body, making it more difficult to wind down.
- **Watching screens** late at night: can cause over-stimulation when you should be winding down; the light from screens disrupts our circadian rhythm.

- **Working** until bedtime (as above).
- **Worrying** about everything you need to do the next day: instead of 'leaving your worries in another room' or on a list.
- **Procrastinating** about even going to bed: watching one more episode, responding to one more email, doing a few household chores, or checking social media, all fight against the body's natural sleep rhythm. Putting off going to bed, because you want to make sure that you are exhausted or because you know you will not get a good sleep perpetuates an out-of-sync routine.

CASE STUDY

Jane used to put off going to bed because she didn't want to be lying awake. She would work or read until 3 am nearly every night, even though she had to be up by 6.30 am each day!

Jane led a very busy and stressful life: with a young family, two jobs, plus various community involvements. Jane knew she needed to get more sleep to function better during the day. And she was consuming a lot of sugary foods during the day to keep herself going. Her pattern of behaviour wasn't logical. Through Brain Coaching, we identified why she was procrastinating. Why was she doing this to herself?

Jane has now established a great bedtime routine: goes to sleep earlier, avoids sugar and alcohol in the evenings, avoids using screens in the evenings, and writes a to-do list. She also repeats a mantra that calms her mind. Jane is now sleeping better and is more productive during the day, (and has reduced her sugar intake).

Anything that will stimulate your system or your brain will keep you from sleeping properly. When you are stimulated, the level of the stress hormone, cortisol, increases in your bloodstream, which then activates adrenalin, leaving you hyped-up, ready to be on alert, ready for fight or flight.

By the end of a busy day, we have dealt with a stream of stressful encounters. It is when we fail to manage the stress in our life that we ruminate over what could have been or should have been done. Worrying about not being able to sleep only adds to this stress, and you are even less likely to fall asleep and stay asleep. This can then become a nightly habit. Thoughts plague your mind, such as:

- How many hours will I get tonight?
- I bet I don't sleep well tonight.
- I'll be hopeless tomorrow if I don't get enough sleep, and then I won't perform well, and my boss will think I'm hopeless, and then I won't get a promotion …

You can see how this sort of thinking is not helpful, possibly adding to your stress levels and making it less likely for you to get a sound sleep. It's important to seek help when we notice we are struggling to manage our responses to everyday stress. This is not an uncommon problem, especially when we consider the many layers of responsibility each of us deals with on a day-to-day basis.

We've all experienced how annoying it is to be woken by the need to go to the toilet. Some bad habits can also lead to the need to empty your bladder in the middle of the night, and now you have established another habit: needing to go to the toilet. Once you are awake, your brain goes over all the things you need to do, didn't do, or didn't say, and so on. *"Where the mind goes - the energy flows," (Ernest Holmes).* If you think about stressful events or things to do, that is where your energy goes; your mind gets busy, making going back to sleep even less likely. As you fight getting back to sleep, thanks to that overactive brain, the body detects a rising anxiety and subtly produces more cortisol, keeping you even more awake. It's important to find a balance between drinking enough to stay hydrated without stimulating a regular need to empty your bladder in the middle of the night. (NB. you can retrain your bladder as well as your brain!)

Pitfalls of Sleeping Tablets

Many people are so desperate for a good night's sleep, they rely on sleeping pills. A study by Scripps Clinic links sleeping pills to a 4.6 times higher risk of death and a significant increase in cancer cases among regular pill users[2]. Many people find that even though they can get to sleep when taking tablets, they still wake up feeling groggy; like having a hangover, and struggle to function efficiently during the day. Many of my clients who had taken sleeping tablets over time were still not getting a refreshing sleep.

Taking sleeping tablets or other supplements, while helpful in the short term, is not a long-term solution. Sleeping pills mask the problem; the real reason you are not able to sleep. They might give you a few good nights' sleep, but in many cases, the effect will wear off and you may feel the need to take more, then more. Relying on sleeping tablets can even lead to people unintentionally overdosing, with terrible results[1].

Always ask your doctor about potential side effects when deciding which sleeping pills to consider taking[3]. Side effects can include:

- ○ Headache.
- ○ Gastrointestinal problems and nausea.

- o Prolonged drowsiness, more so with drugs that help you stay asleep.
- o Dizziness or light-headedness, which may lead to falls.
- o Severe allergic reaction.
- o Sleep-related behaviours, such as driving or eating when not fully awake.
- o Daytime memory and performance problems.

BUT!!! – I hear you say …

"I absolutely have to check my emails and social media feeds before I go to bed!"
I know how tempting it is to do that one quick check, but before you know it, you're up all night. Let's try to break that habit, right now! Try putting your device in a bedside drawer or out of reach. Building new habits takes practice.

"We always have a big meal at night."
Maybe you can explain to the cook why you want to eat smaller meals at night – make it a family/household mission. Small adjustments make a big difference if you are suffering from poor sleep.

"I enjoy my glasses of wine every night."
Try substituting wine for something non-alcoholic later in the day and look forward to better sleep, a clearer head, and not having to get up to go to the toilet at night.

"I can only exercise strenuously in the evenings."
Sometimes it is just more important to prioritise sleep. When you value your quality of sleep, you will find alternative solutions.

"Having coffee late into the afternoon and evening is essential to my creativity and productivity."
Getting off the caffeine round-about can be challenging – but surviving on compromised sleep when that caffeine keeps you awake at night can be harder to recover from in the long run.

"I need that sleeping tablet!!"
Logically, you know pills lose their impact and still make you feel groggy the next day. When you don't take it, your body can adjust to using fewer addictive alternatives. Brain Coaching can help you develop strategies to improve your sleeping habits.

"I put off going to bed because I want to make sure I am super-tired."
It sounds like a good theory but may only add to your stress. Staying up late involves fighting against your natural sleep rhythms. Notice when you start to yawn – that's the perfect time to start your sleep routine.

"I put off going to sleep because that's the only time I get to myself. That is my me time."
When 'me time' cuts into sleep time, your choice may begin to affect your health.

Chapter Summary

People develop habits that are not conducive to good sleep for many reasons. It takes an individual approach to solve the problem. Every person is different, and everyone has a unique set of problems and issues. That's why it is crucial to identify the real reason for insomnia and develop strategies just for you. The first step is to ascertain whether the reason for the disruptive habit is environmental, medical, physiological, or emotional. Subsequent treatments and therapies will then depend on the original cause.

These bad habits may be pleasurable at the time - drinking alcohol, exercising, or being on social media late in the evening - but in the long term, is the momentary pleasure worth the risks that lack of sleep brings to your life? It doesn't mean that you have to give up all your pleasures, it just means that maybe you could indulge in them at a different time of day or come up with healthier alternatives.

Brain Coaching can help you uncover the real social or emotional reason you are not sleeping, and then help you develop strategies to overcome poor habits that will suit you and your lifestyle.

Taking advantage of the brain's plasticity makes it possible to change your habits and ways of thinking, create new, good habits, and start sleeping better.

If you have realised that one or more bad habits could be contributing to your sleep issues, you can try changing just one of these habits today. For example, give up coffee in the evenings; or just do gentle exercises before bed, rather than strenuous exercise; or turn off your screens one hour before bed. You will need to practise any new habit for a few weeks to change poor habits into good habits. We can all make excuses for why we let ourselves get into these bad habits. Now is the time to do something about it. You are worth the effort.

CHAPTER 4

Environmental Conditions for Optimal Sleep

"My bed is my magical place where I suddenly remember all the things I was supposed to do!" (Anonymous)

An environment conducive to sleep centres around the physical set-up of your room, bed, and bedding. A room that is too hot, too cold, too noisy, too bright, constantly disrupted by other people (snoring partner or people you are caring for, or noisy neighbours), or has uncomfortable bedding will play a part[1].

In your quest to get a good night's sleep, you must firstly address any physical or environmental problems. If sleep is still an issue after sorting your physical environment, then you will need to look at other possible issues, such as medical or emotional issues.

Keeping a sleep diary will help identify patterns or issues that are influencing your insomnia. Once you can identify something that needs changing, change one thing at a time.

Let's look at particular environmental factors that influence great sleep:
Room temperature: Your body temperature drops during the night so you need to keep warm, or feeling cold may wake you up. The ideal room temperature should be about 16-18^{0}C. If the room is too warm or bedding too hot (for some over 24^{0}C), you will become restless. Have you ever had to stick your feet out from under the covers during the night? If the room or bedding is too cool (for some below 12^{0}C), it may be difficult to get to sleep and stay asleep, because you can't warm up. Children and older people may need slightly warmer temperatures or bedding for a night of better sleep.

Bed, Bedding and Pillows: Lightweight bedding for summer (with an extra blanket kept nearby), and warmer bedding for winter is ideal. As for the actual bed – everyone is different, so it will pay to thoroughly test and find the right mattress for you and your partner. Old, lumpy, sagging beds will not suit your posture or sleep. A bed that is too hard may cause pressure points on your hips and shoulders and you'll be too uncomfortable for deep sleep.

Your preferred sleeping position will influence the type of pillow you should choose.

People who sleep on their stomachs should choose a flat, soft pillow or no pillow at all. People who sleep on their side should have a pillow that supports the head and neck and provides proper spine alignment. People who sleep on their back should have a pillow with medium support to cradle the head. Pillow architecture is also significant – too high or too hard can cause neck aches, too low or too soft can bend the neck the opposite way. It is worthwhile investing in a good pillow, rather than a cheaper one that will lose shape in a matter of weeks or months.

Pillow quality is an important consideration. A synthetic pillow has a life of up to two years, while a natural fibre-filled pillow (feathers, down, natural fibres) has a life of up to ten years. In his book 'The Barefoot Investor', Scott Pape says that a good quality pillow is one of the best investments you can make[2]!

The material used in the filling of a pillow is also important. The aim is to draw heat away from the head during the night. Pillows that allow the head to overheat can have a negative impact on sleep quality and continuity. Pillows filled with natural fibres are usually better at drawing heat away from the head. These days, many pillows are made of synthetic material. Of course, people with allergies should consider pillows made with hypoallergenic materials. Soft, moldable down-filled pillows are another option.

No matter how good your pillow is, it won't last a lifetime. When pillows start losing their shape, it is usually time to replace them. As pillows age, they collect allergy triggers, dead skin cells and dust mites. Most pillows can be machine washed, however, check the label first. Wash pillows a few times a year to clean out dust, mites, allergy triggers, and grime, which can be the reasons some people are kept awake. Pillow protectors can help extend a pillow's lifespan. To check if your pillow needs replacing, fold it in half and see if it springs back to its original shape. If it doesn't, then your pillow needs replacing.

Weighted Blankets: These blankets have glass, metal or plastic weights sewn into them. *"The feeling is like giving yourself a hug,"* said a client who uses one. People have been helped to get better sleep by using weighted blankets. They feel it helps reduce their stress levels. The promoters of weighted blankets say that the gentle pressure of the extra weight induces a sense of calm, similar to how a baby swaddled in a blanket is provided a sense of security. This sense of calm can help to reduce cortisol (the stress hormone) and encourage the production of melatonin (the sleep hormone) and serotonin (the relaxing hormone). Although there are few research studies on their value to improve sleep, Choice Magazine did a consumer survey, and many consumers found weighted blankets were "*nice, but not worth the money*" [3]. There is a warning that some people with medical problems and young children should not have weighted blankets because it may impede their breathing while sleeping. Best to consult your doctor first.

Noise: If, after trying everything to reduce noise in your household during sleeping hours, there are still noises beyond your control, you may need to invest in double-glazing, heavy curtains or earplugs. Some people prefer 'white noise' rather than the noise of traffic, trains, neighbours etc. White noise can include the sound of a fan, meditation music or ocean sounds. Other people can even go to sleep listening to the sound of a dishwasher (their equivalent of white noise!) White noise is constant - there are no harsh or loud jumps in sound decibels. This method is especially useful when travelling and staying in different environments. For example, the constant noise of the air-conditioner can drown out the noise of passing vehicles or rowdy neighbours. The white noise from an untuned radio station, or a white noise app, has been found to help many of my clients. Another alternative is ASMR (autonomous sensory meridian response). This is a lesser-known method for distracting and relaxing the brain into sleep. It works for some people, while others have said it had no effect. You will need to try for yourself to see what works for you. There are many sources available online.

Some people listen to quiet talkback radio in the early hours, which puts them to sleep!

Light: The intensity of light in the bedroom affects our circadian rhythm. The presence of light alerts our brain that daylight is here, and that it is time to start the day. Whereas when it is dark, our bodies release melatonin, a hormone that helps us relax. Turn all gadget lights off or cover them up. Outdoor lights can be intrusive, so use blackout blinds or curtains if possible, or use an eye mask. Masks may seem awkward at first but believe me, they come in handy when you are travelling! Some people have unplugged everything in their motel room to help reduce intermittent noise and intrusive standby lights or pegged curtains to minimise outdoor light seeping into the room.

Electronic devices: The noise and light emitting from these devices will disrupt sleep. The stimulation to the brain from playing games, sending work emails, or watching or reading items on these devices at night will play havoc with sleep patterns. Your bed is not the place for this type of stimulation. If your brain is over-stimulated right before turning off your device, it may be difficult to get to sleep and stay asleep.

A tip from a client: she puts her phone or alarm clock out of reach of the bed, to remove the temptation to keep looking at the time.

People: You may eliminate noise and light, but it is difficult to eliminate people from your night's sleep. That person may be your co-sleeper, someone you are caring for who may have disruptive patterns, or noisy neighbours who have different sleeping patterns to you. If your sleep is disrupted because you are caring for someone who wakes during the night (a baby or a person with an illness or special needs), then you need to get back to sleep easily. If your co-sleeping partner is disrupting your sleep, then you may need to negotiate solutions that will suit you both. You may need to consult a family counsellor if you cannot come up with your own solutions, or if earplugs are not enough! Alternative arrangements may need to be carefully negotiated. If the problem is coming from outside your home, you may need to consult a landlord arbitrator, or report extremely noisy neighbours to local authorities (especially if their animals are keeping you awake, and probably keeping other people awake too). If, after addressing the suggestions in this section, you are struggling to develop your own solutions, Brain Coaching can help build confidence and skills to help approach difficult conversations. The conversation usually goes well when you are calm and have all your facts or reasons in order, and you can outline a satisfactory outcome for both parties. It's called, "How to Present an Argument and not Lose Friends!" I show people how to do this in my workshops. It is incredible how easy it is once you start practicing.

Animals: Your pets, or neighbours' pets, can disrupt good sleep. It is essential to create an amenable animal routine at bedtime before poor habits take hold of your night's sleep. There are tips on the internet about how to train your pet to behave in the middle of the night. If pets are disruptive, it's important to find out the reason they are being a nuisance in the middle of the night or early morning, and deal with that first. Some tips for training your pet include: providing active play just before bedtime so that they don't feel lonely, and to tire them out. Or leaving food and water for them during the night, so they are not waking you for this reason. If pets sleep on your bed and wake you by moving around or touching you, you need to decide which you want more - the animal's company, or better sleep. Yes, you can retrain your pet into suitable night-time habits. It takes patience and consistency. Part of the retraining includes ignoring unwanted behaviour, feeding at a different time, and/or giving attention to them prior to bed. Whatever you do, do not reward bad behaviour, reward good behaviour.

Neighbours' pets are a different matter, and any issues will require negotiation and/or mediation.

BUT!!! - I hear you say …

"My neighbour is unapproachable, (or too nice), I can't raise the issue with them."

The alternative is to move house! Or come up with a creative solution. Negotiate or bring in arbitration. A Brain Coaching session can help you determine which way you would feel more comfortable approaching the issue.

"My partner is too sensitive, or argumentative, or works too hard. I can't disrupt their sleep or upset them, even if they are the one who is snoring or restless or has different sleeping patterns to me."

There are methods that can help strengthen your confidence to broach sensitive issues in a calm, relaxed way.

"My pet has a mind of its own."

Sometimes it can take outside help to assist you with your commitment and persistence. You can retrain your pet or think of alternative solutions. You still love your pet; you are trying to work out what is going to be best for both of you.

"There are noises and lights from traffic."

Apart from moving house, you could move to a different room, install double glazing, or thick curtains. Alternatively, use earplugs, or listen to white noise. In Brain Coaching sessions, we uncover your preferred strategy for dealing with the noise. Intervention can also help you accept the situation, in the case of traffic noise. Many people who live near a railway line can sleep right through the night!

"I can't afford new bedding."

Think of new bedding as an investment. The better sleep you have, the more productive you become.

Brain Coaching will help improve your mindset when dealing with difficult people. It will help improve your motivation, confidence, and persistence to solve problems that keep all involved happy. Together, we develop your own strategies to help reinforce a new way of thinking, making it easier for you to follow through with your plans. Brain Coaching focuses on logical solutions rather than allowing emotions, like frustration or fear, to take over. If you get a good night's sleep, you are more likely to handle what the day brings from neighbours, partners, or animals, in a more relaxed, less emotional way.

Chapter Summary

Once you realise that your sleeping problem may stem from your environment, you can do something about it, before the sleeping problem becomes a persistent habit. Solutions to improve your sleeping environment may be relatively simple, but you just haven't considered them yet, or you're not yet motivated to attend to them. For example, moving your bedroom to the rear of the house away from traffic noise, or adjusting the bedroom temperature or wearing earplugs, are relatively simple, inexpensive solutions. Other solutions could be more expensive or complicated: buying a new bed, installing double-glazing, or dealing with a snoring partner. You may need to weigh the pros and cons to make a choice that works. When the problem calls for extra support, Brain Coaching can help you sort through what you really want to implement in your life, and then helps boost your motivation and confidence to see things through. The result may mean that you learn to put up with a difficult situation/environment, if you can't change it, AND be able to get yourself back to sleep if you do wake up.

Imagine nestling into a comfortable bed, with the appropriate lighting and temperature and minimal noise. You deserve to have the right setting that is conducive for good sleep.

Handy Checklist of Environmental Conditions Conducive to a Good Night's Sleep:

☐ Dark room/heavy curtains/minimal or no internal lights.
☐ Room temperature - ideally 16-18°C.
☐ Bedding appropriate for each individual's needs – comfort and temperature.
☐ Reduce noise or use white noise.
☐ Sort out disruptive people/animals.
☐ Avoid electronic devices in the bedroom.

How do you score?

CHAPTER 5

Physiological Issues Affecting Sleeping Habits

"Sleep is the 3rd pillar of good health,
the other two are diet and exercise."
(Harvard School of Sleep Medicine).

Definition: *Physiology is the science of life. This branch of biology aims to understand the mechanisms of living things, from the basis of cell function at the ionic and molecular level to the integrated behaviour of the whole body and the influence of the external environment. Research in physiology helps us to understand how the body works in health and how it responds and adapts to the challenges of everyday life; it also helps us to determine what goes wrong in disease, facilitating the development of new treatments and guidelines for maintaining human and animal health. (https:// www.physoc.org/explore-physiology/what-is-physiology/)*

Physiology refers simply to how all the systems in our body react and work together, allowing us to function as well as we can. Our physiology is sensitive to factors which affect our sleep. The interaction between our body's digestive, hormonal, nervous and circulation systems helps us regulate our sleep patterns.

For example:

- Different levels of light affect our internal biological clock.
- You may have experienced that heavy, sleepy feeling after eating a large, indulgent meal – our body is working so hard on digesting, there's little energy for anything else!
- Have you felt the after-effects of an extended, sedentary trip, we think of as 'jet lag', and how it may take days for your body to return to its regular routine? The effects of changing time zones impacts our physiology.
- Illness can affect our sleep patterns. With some illnesses we can sleep for days, while with others we can't sleep at all.

There are other factors that can affect each of our physiological systems and impact our sleep that are well within our scope to influence. We can implement 'body hacks' and improve our sleep patterns if we are willing to persist and create new or improved sleeping habits.

We have the power to adjust detrimental lifestyle habits before our bodies require medical intervention – for sleep disorders or any other health issue. YOU have influence over your own body to improve your sleep patterns, and if you need motivation to implement some of the physiological hacks mentioned in this chapter, Brain Coaching can help you succeed.

Problems affecting our physiological processes can often be relatively easy to overcome, with just a few tweaks. The first step is gaining awareness of the issue and what you can do about it. As desperate as it may feel, when running on little or no sleep, you are not entirely powerless or without hope. In this chapter, we will look at the most relevant physiological factors impacting sleep and learn some easy body hacks that can positively influence our own body's function in order to have better sleep. **Let your body help you!**

Three researchers won the Nobel Prize for Physiology or Medicine in 2017 for their work on the circadian rhythm and its subsequent effect on the physiology of humans.

The winning researchers were - Jeffrey C. Hall, Michael Rosbash and Michael W. Young.

"Their discoveries explain how plants, animals and humans adapt their biological rhythm to synchronize with the Earth's revolutions." (https://www.nobelprize.org/prizes/medicine/2017/press-release).

Circadian Rhythm (CR)

Illness, stress or bad habits can impact our circadian rhythm, affecting our well-being, and particularly the ability to sleep well. Going to bed in the early morning hours, eating big meals late at night, keeping lights on past bedtime, shift work, or jet lag are all disruptive to our circadian rhythm.

Among other functions, our circadian rhythm regulates nightly body temperature. It cools us down when we are tired and then warms us up when it's time to wake. If we are overheated or too cold while we sleep, we will wake up out of sync with our cycle, resulting in disturbed sleep habits.

The amount of light in our bedroom can affect our circadian rhythm and put our sleep out of order. Light suppresses melatonin (the sleep hormone), which helps let our body know that it is time to sleep. If there is too much light when we are supposed to be sleeping, it will be more challenging to fall asleep.

Different foods can provide melatonin, which helps us feel sleepy by bedtime, keeping the circadian rhythm in good order. Bananas, warm milk, almonds, fish, spinach, chickpeas, yeast extract, kiwi fruit, and vitamin C can all provide melatonin to support your circadian rhythm.

Meditation and deep breathing can also help keep the circadian rhythm on track. Deep breathing helps oxygenate our blood, which is good for brain function and also slows our heart rate, reducing stress. Exposure to daily sunlight, especially in the early morning, is also very beneficial.

Gut/Brain connection

The gut covers the digestive tract from the stomach to the bowel, including the nervous and other systems. There have been many studies looking into the gut/brain connection. Some scientists are even calling the gut our second brain! What happens in the gut impacts our brain and how we feel; and what happens in the brain can influence our emotions and impact the gut. Have you ever felt so nervous or anxious that you experienced 'butterflies', a churning stomach, or even diarrhea?

CASE STUDY

I have a few clients who suffered from Irritable Bowel Syndrome or diarrhea due to stress, which disrupted their sleep. Once we overcame the trigger for the original stress, these clients devised their own strategies to deal with that trigger and develop coping methods that reduced their stress. Not only did their IBS go away, but they also started sleeping better. They shared that they couldn't believe how good they felt!

The gut/brain connection is significant to overall health as it affects our immune system and emotional well-being. There is now evidence that the micro bacteria in your gut also influence sleep patterns. These bacteria can impact the hormones related to sleep - serotonin and melatonin[1].

There are simple ways to improve your gut bacteria to get better sleep: you can increase your dietary fibre content, and include fermented foods, prebiotics, and probiotics (see box for explanation), reduce processed foods and eat earlier in the evening.

The gut's bacteria also influence hormone levels related to feelings of satiety, the 'full' feeling you notice after eating a meal. Leptin is the hormone that tells us when we are full. People who produce less leptin sometimes don't know when to stop eating. Lack of sleep can impact the level of this hormone, so sleep deprivation can indirectly lead to overeating, not because we are making poor choices and have less self-control, but because we are tired. A lack of sleep also affects another hormone related to eating and appetite called, ghrelin. This hormone tells us when we are hungry. If we have too much of this hormone, we eat more because we are feeling hungry.

Prebiotics and Probiotics

"A prebiotic is a type of fibre (but not all fibre is prebiotic). To be classified as a prebiotic, the fibre must pass through the gastrointestinal tract undigested and stimulate certain 'good' bacteria's growth and/or activity in the large intestine."[2]

See Table 1 below for examples of food that are naturally high in prebiotics.

Probiotics are different in that they contain live bacteria or yeasts, which add to your gut's population of healthy microbes.[3] Probiotics can be eaten as food or supplements. Yoghurt is the most common probiotic. Other bacteria-fermented foods containing probiotics are sauerkraut, kombucha, and kimchi. Probiotic supplements contain live organisms. A dietitian can advise you on food sources for prebiotics and probiotics.

Gut Biome

"The gut biome is the collection of microorganisms that live in the digestive tract," British Medical Journal

Health benefits of digesting prebiotics include; improved gut microbiota, increased absorption of essential minerals, protection against colon cancer, improved blood glucose and insulin levels; protection against intestinal infections; and improved or reduced progress of some inflammatory conditions.

Maintaining a healthy gut biome involves increasing the number of good bacteria by eating prebiotics and, ideally, probiotics. Reducing the amount of processed food, sugar and fat, and increasing the amount and diversity of high-fibre food keeps your gut biome happy.

Table 1. Foods naturally high in prebiotics. (Courtesy Monash University Gastroenterology Dept):

Vegetables	Jerusalem artichokes, chicory, garlic, onion, leek, shallots, spring onion, asparagus, beetroot, fennel bulb, green peas, snow peas, sweetcorn, savoy cabbage
Legumes	Chickpeas, lentils, red kidney beans, baked beans, soybeans
Fruit	Custard apples, nectarines, white peaches, persimmon, tamarillo, watermelon, rambutan, grapefruit, pomegranate. Dried fruit (dates, figs)
Bread/ Cereals	Barley, rye bread, rye crackers, pasta, gnocchi, couscous, wheat bran, wheat bread, oats
Nuts	Cashews, pistachio nuts

When there is an imbalance in the gut/brain connection, the result of lack of sleep and/or a weakened immune system, we can become vulnerable to diseases, including cancer, gastric esophogeal reflux disease (GERD), irritable bowel, Crohn's, and ulcerative colitis. Sleep-deprived people seem to have a higher incidence of these diseases[4].

GERD (American) or GORD (English) stands for Gastric Esophageal/Oesophageal Reflux Disease. People can also suffer from Silent Reflux (laryngopharyngeal reflux or LPR). Over the past few years, I have noticed that many of my sleep clients also have gastric reflux and are taking Nexium (or similar) for it.

Gastric Reflux is also known as heartburn. The research shows that stress and lack of sleep contribute to gastric reflux. The difference between GERD and Silent reflux is the lack of noticeable symptoms of heartburn when you have silent reflux. Both conditions seem to be worse at night, when lying down. Silent Reflux symptoms include blocked nasal passages at night, and a feeling of a lump in your throat, where you feel the need to be constantly trying to clear your throat. During the day, the symptoms seem to clear up. This subtle condition can lead to disturbed sleep, as you can't breathe properly when you feel your nose is blocked, and you are persistently trying to cough up a lump of phlegm.

For both GERD and LRP, stress disrupts the balance of acid in the digestive tract, but GERD gives you the feeling of heartburn as the reflux comes back up into the larynx and throat area when you are lying down. There is a bidirectional effect: poor sleep leads to a more stressful life, and more stress can lead to stomach acid coming back up, leading to poor sleep. There is a combination of two recommended treatments:

1. Decrease stress, and
2. Treat the reflux with either pharmaceuticals and/or physical adjustments, like avoiding spicy foods and alcohol within 3 hours of bedtime or sleeping with your head at a higher incline.

The outcome should cause better sleep, less stress, as well as a clearer throat and nasal passages. The understanding of this condition has been a revelation for some of my clients who had never made a connection between constantly having to clear their throat and having poor sleep. The two conditions were not necessarily linked.

Other studies have found that an improved gut biome equals improved mood and a reduction in sleep disorders.

The gut/brain connection works in both directions. Brain activity can affect the biome in your gut. If you are stressed and not sleeping well, your gut health will be affected. Reducing stress will improve your gut biome. If you are stressed, you need to pinpoint your stressors. Deep breathing or meditation are recommended to help decrease stress and will work immediately. Long-term strategies for reducing stress will need to be explored and other parts of your life will need to be considered. Brain Coaching is the perfect tool for exploring options for you.

Diagram of cycle of improved gut biome.

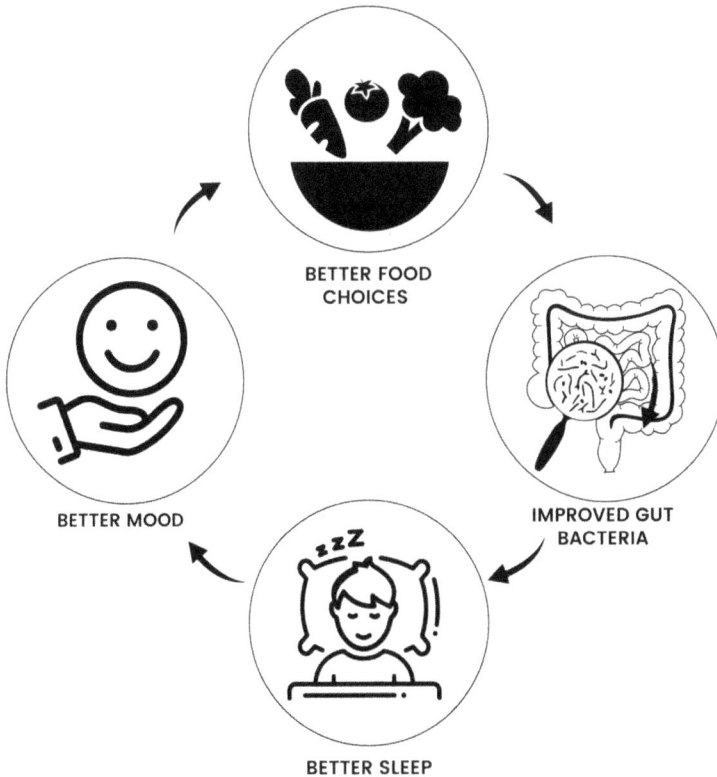

BETTER FOOD CHOICES

IMPROVED GUT BACTERIA

BETTER SLEEP

BETTER MOOD

It is worth trying a probiotic or increasing prebiotic foods in your diet for a few weeks to see if they work for you. If you are still not sleeping properly, then a session with your Brain Coach, to further investigate why, may be just what you need.

Vagus nerve and its role in sleep patterns:
The vagus nerve is the longest nerve in the body. It connects the brain to the gut and other vital organs, like the heart and lungs. When our vagus nerve is toned, we enjoy a reduced heart rate, lower blood pressure, better digestion (less gut churning) and better hormone balance.

The vagus nerve is part of the parasympathetic nervous system (PSNS)[5], otherwise known as the 'rest and digest' system. The PSNS is involved in regulating our automatic bodily functions like heartbeat, breathing and digestion, even while we are sleeping.

When our vagus nerve is in-tune, we feel more positive, and the more positive we feel in both mind and body, the more our vagus nerve will be in balance.

Improving our vagal responses can improve many aspects of our mind and body. We can improve our response to stress and recover more quickly from illness or injury. At the other end of the 'rest and digest' scale is 'fight or flight' mode. When we are in fight or flight, our body prepares us to do just that! When we are in this heightened state of reaction, we find it difficult to switch off and sleep peacefully.

It is possible to stimulate your vagus nerve and see an improvement in the above functions. You can buy an electronic stimulator that plugs onto your earlobe, or you can do it manually. Here are some easy ways to improve the tone of your vagus nerve[6]:

- Exposure to cold temperature – have a cold shower for 30 seconds; or place your hands or face into ice-cold water.
- Diaphragm breathing - deep, slow 'belly' breathing.
- Laughing, singing, humming, chanting, gargling to stimulate vocal cords.
- Probiotics.
- Meditation and/or yoga.
- Massaging the vagus nerve on the right side of your neck, near the carotid sinus.
- Exercise.

Engaging the vagus nerve, with its connections to the major organs of the body, helps to calm the body after stress, bringing us back into balance, promoting sleep. It takes us out of constant flight or fight mode, and the feeling of being switched on all day and all night.

If our vagus nerve is out of tone, we will feel wired or less at ease, less able to cope with everyday happenings. When we feel less at ease, we find ourselves increasingly self-critical, self-berating and negative self-talk can become a habit that keeps looping in our brain, suppressing the vagus nerve, possibly leading to depression and poor sleep patterns.

A study by Breit et al. (2018) conducted quite an in-depth trial and reported on how nutrition, mindfulness activities, and vagus nerve stimulation all impact our well-being in a positive way[7]. De-stressing, relaxing, hormone regulation and psychotherapy can all lead to better well-being, a healthier body and better sleep.

Exercise – timing and quality

Adequate exercise is important for good sleep patterns. It helps reduce the severity of Sleep Disordered Breathing (SDB). Obstructive sleep apnoea (OSA) is the most common type of SDB. A meta-analysis by Kline (2014) found that exercise training reduced OSA severity even without people losing weight[8]. They found that twelve weeks of moderate-intensity aerobic and resistance exercise resulted in a 25% reduction in the severity of Sleep Apnoea. Exercise training also *"led to better sleep and improved daytime functioning (e.g., quality of life, depressive symptoms, vigour, fatigue)"*.[9]

Timing of your exercise can be important for improving sleep patterns, either letting your body know when to rev up or to prepare for sleep. Along with lighter dinners, dimming lighting, adjusting temperature, avoiding stimulating games or working late at night; the timing of physical activities is critical when preparing your body for sleep.

Too much vigorous exercise late at night stimulates blood flow and increases endorphins, making it harder for the brain and body to settle. Sleep researchers have stated that morning exercise is better for most people, but if this isn't possible, exercising at least two hours before bedtime will allow your body and your hormones time to settle. This situation is similar for people who have just come off shift work – it is hard to go to sleep straight away, and shift workers need a few hours between work and sleep to allow the sleep cycle to adjust. I know people who exercise vigorously at nighttime and then struggle to calm down enough to get to sleep. Together, we worked on some alternative strategies they were happy to implement to get a whole night's sleep.

Exercising raises body temperature, which is another reason to give your body time to settle before bedtime, allowing your temperature to drop.

Researchers at the Johns Hopkins Centre have recommended gentle exercise after the evening meal, like a stroll, or mild yoga. This will also aid digestion before bed. They add that gentle exercise promotes slow wave or deep sleep. Gentle exercise, *"stabilises your mood and relaxes the mind and is also important in obtaining a good night's sleep."*[10].

I recommend that thirty minutes of exercise per day, at least two hours before bed, is best for overall health and improved sleep. The timing of exercise, whether morning, afternoon or evening, is up to the individual, and how it suits their lifestyle, as long as it is at least two hours prior to bedtime.

Researchers from the Sleep Foundation (2020) have found that exercise (if the timing is right), can be as effective as sleeping tablets[11]. Your core body temperature rises during exercise, then drops when it is time for bed. It brings your body back into the circadian rhythm, which is what some pharmaceuticals try to do.

The endorphins released during exercise can also help ease feelings of anxiety and depression. If you exercise, this could be another reason you may not need pharmaceuticals. Lack of exercise has also been a predictor of insomnia. Many people who don't exercise also don't sleep well. This is a bidirectional relationship – you are tired, so you don't exercise; if you don't exercise, you have poor sleep and are tired the next day, so you feel even less likely to exercise.

"Instead of waiting to feel good to exercise, go out and exercise and then you will feel good."

People who exercise get better sleep, are less stressed, make better choices, are more productive, and are more pleasant to be around. Not only do their lives improve, but so do their relationships with people around them – their family, work colleagues, their community. By extension, daily exercise leads to fewer health problems and less dependence on the health system.

Nutrition, Mealtimes and Helpful Foods

As with the timing of exercise, the timing of the evening meal or night-time snacking is also important for getting the body ready for sleep. Food digestion involves the release of insulin and other digestive hormones, which are linked to the proper function of our circadian rhythm. It is recommended to finish heavy meals at least three hours before bedtime. This allows the body time to digest the food and also provides time for the hormones to come back into balance before the circadian rhythm is disrupted, and sleep gets later and later. It is important to allow sufficient fasting time between dinner and breakfast (that is why it is called breakfast – you are breaking the fast) and allow enough time for restorative sleep. Not to mention, the physical discomfort of eating a large meal prior to bedtime keeping you awake, with a higher likelihood of indigestion, further compounding your sleep dilemma.

There seems to be some conjecture amongst sleep experts whether the food we eat impacts the quality and quantity of our sleep, or whether our quality and quantity of sleep impacts what we eat. For instance, whether we are too tired to make the right food choices, or do our food choices affect our sleep?

Many studies have examined the impact of different foods and their effects on sleep. One mega-study by Binks et al., (2020) identified over 2500 articles concerning sleep and diet[12]. Their review of these studies found that a diet with little or no tryptophan led to increased sleep disruptions. Tryptophan is an amino acid that is involved in the production of melatonin (the main hormone helping us sleep). It can be found in turkey meat and milk products. Carbohydrates also have a role in producing tryptophan. Perhaps we need to be wary of limiting carbohydrates too drastically. Scientists are still researching the benefits of eating too many carbohydrates or no carbohydrates at nighttime.

Research indicates that low Glycaemic Index (GI) carbohydrates are better at producing tryptophan. Whereas high GI carbohydrates, refined carbs like sugar and white flour products, can lead to insomnia. One of my clients has definitely noticed this: *"When I eat sweet things at night, I have noticed that I might only get two hours sleep. That is when I use the Brain Coaching techniques and my sleep improves again."* Some people can get back to sleep by eating something, as long as it is not refined carbohydrates!

"Carbohydrates have a big role to play in treating insomnia," said Vlahoyiannis et al., (2021), in their meta-analysis of twenty-seven trials, on the effects of carbohydrates on sleep[13]. The body needs carbohydrates for the energy they supply which helps brain function. Low GI is better than high GI, as low GI foods have more fibre and nutrients and last longer in our system than highly processed carbohydrates. High GI foods result in sugar spikes in our systems, which can wake us at 3am - then cortisol is subsequently released, making it difficult to get back to sleep[14].

Other nutrients which can influence sleep:

Zinc helps to increase the production of serotonin. Oysters, red meat, legumes, almonds, walnuts or zinc supplements can work, but they will have a bigger impact on sleep if your body is already low on zinc.

Vitamin B6 can help with our sleep patterns, especially when combined with foods that have an antioxidant effect. Good sources of B6 are: tuna, salmon, chickpeas, poultry, dark leafy greens, bananas, papaya, oranges, rock melon, eggs.

Phlorotannins are antioxidants commonly found in brown seaweed. They have been shown to significantly decrease sleep latency (the time it takes to fall asleep) and increase NREM sleep. In a 2018 research trial, the sleep-promoting effects of phlorotannin supplements at 500 mg/day were comparable to those of the positive control, diazepam (valium) at 6 mg/day. In this randomised, double-blind, placebo-controlled clinical trial of 20 volunteers, phlorotannin supplements significantly decreased wakefulness after sleep onset compared to the placebo[15].

Phytonutrients obtained from tart cherries have been found to aid insomnia by improving the production of melatonin and serotonin. They also have antioxidant and anti-inflammatory properties[16].

St Onge (2016), and Lin (2011), both looked into the effect of kiwi fruit on sleep problems and found that kiwi fruit aided sleep thanks to its antioxidant and folate content, as well as increasing serotonin levels[17]. Folate deficiency is associated with insomnia and restless leg syndrome.

Magnesium and fatty acids help to relieve insomnia and are found in almonds and walnuts. They help reduce inflammation and cortisol levels while increasing melatonin levels, making them more conducive to better sleep. Many of my clients say that they have used magnesium, in either a lotion, bath salts, or tablet form, to help them sleep. Some people had better results than others.

Fish which are high in Omega3 oils also contain vitamin D, which can improve sleep.

It has been recommended that a small amount of glycine supplement taken daily may aid sleep patterns and be a harmless alternative to sleeping pills. Glycine is an amino acid that benefits many parts of our physiology. It has a calming effect on the brain, and can reduce core body temperature, making sleep more likely to happen. 3mg per day is considered a safe amount to take as a supplement, although it is also found in different foods like - meat, fish, dairy products, and legumes[18].

Summary of foods that have been found to relieve insomnia:

Food	Nutrient
Turkey meat, dairy products, low GI carbohydrates (e.g., whole grains, brown rice, etc)	Tryptophan
Oysters, red meat, legumes	Zinc
Almonds, walnuts	Zinc, magnesium and fatty acids
Tuna, salmon, chickpeas, poultry, dark leafy greens, bananas, papaya, oranges, rock melon, eggs	Vitamin B6
Seaweed	Phlorotannins
Tart cherries	Phytonutrients
Kiwi fruit	Folate
Fish, seafood, nuts, seeds and plant oils	Omega-3, fatty acids, and Vitamin D
Mushrooms	Vitamin D
Meat, fish, dairy, legumes or supplement form	Glycine

Nutrients from whole, real foods are considered to be of greater benefit to sleep than nutrients derived from supplements. This is mainly because of their fibre content - they make you feel fuller and last longer in your system.

Some foods to avoid consuming late at night include those containing caffeine, alcohol, and heavy, fatty, or spicy food. Foods (or meals) high in fat and high GI carbohydrates consumed late at night can affect your sleep by interfering with the production of sleep-inducing hormones. This can have a subsequent impact on the Central Nervous System (CNS) and the metabolic system, which then influences the production of the hormones, ghrelin and leptin. These hormones influence how respectively full or hungry you feel. Feeling hungry can lead to sleep disruption, waking you up, feeling alert in the middle of the night, when you should be feeling sleepy.

All the above dietary suggestions are helpful, less expensive, and have less side effects than pharmaceutical solutions to treat insomnia. And isn't it great that these suggestions also follow the guidelines for healthy dietary advice?

Hydration and Sleep

Sleep and hydration are the key elements for beauty sleep! However, there is a fine line between being suitably hydrated for sound sleep and being over-hydrated, leading to the need for urinating at night, waking us up, and causing trouble getting back to sleep. Not enough fluids during the day can cause dehydration, which disrupts our sleep patterns. Researchers have conducted trials that suggest that lack of sleep may lead to waking up feeling dehydrated, and that being dehydrated can lead to a more wakeful night[19]. Not only does urination cause water loss from the body, but the body also loses water when breathing out (respiration), even while sleeping. If sleep is interrupted, this can impact the body clock, then the production of another hormone (vasopressin) involved in keeping our water levels in balance can be thrown out of kilter. The trick here is to drink enough water during the day so that our bodies are sufficiently hydrated to last through the night, but not be over-hydrated so that we need to get up to urinate.

It is possible to retrain your bladder to reduce the urge to urinate (as long as there are no medical reasons for this issue). If you must go, then try not to wake up completely by turning on all the lights or checking your phone for messages! Make the trip to the toilet as unobtrusive as possible, so that you are more likely to get back to sleep on your return. Retraining your bladder involves putting off going to the bathroom for as long as you can each night. It will seem impossible at first, but gradually, you will last longer and longer each night before needing the toilet.

CASE STUDY

I have had clients who used to go to the toilet around 4-5 times per night. It only took a few nights of retraining their bladder, and their brain, to convince them they didn't really need to go that often. They now tell me they sleep longer and more deeply than they ever did. As a bonus to sleeping better, they also say they are less stressed the next day.

Another reason to avoid caffeine and alcohol just prior to bedtime is that both cause dehydration. Being dehydrated during the night can also be the reason for headaches, muscle cramps, or a dry nose and mouth, which can lead to a wakeful night. Avoid becoming overheated during the night and sweating excess fluid – adjust your environment to suit.

Please see your doctor if you are concerned about dehydration or hydration issues affecting your sleep.

Obesity

Weight gain can lead to sleep problems. Fat can build up along the airways, at the base of the tongue and around the neck, making it harder to breathe[20]. Along with extra weight pressing on the neck or the lungs, causing a reduction in lung volume, airways can collapse and problems occur with breathing, like snoring or sleep apnoea, and hypoventilation. Being overweight can impact our sleep because it impacts our breathing mechanism.

Snoring occurs when airways are obstructed, and sleep apnoea occurs when the airways are so blocked that breathing pauses, and people constantly wake up because they can't breathe. They find themselves 'gasping for air'. Snoring in children is usually due to enlarged tonsils or adenoids and may need to be seen to by a doctor.

If you are having trouble with any of the above but feel you can't change your habits: can't wear the CPAP machine's mask, or can't lose weight, then Brain Coaching is an option that can unlock emotional blockages and redirect your mindset. The logical side of you knows that serious health and relationship issues will arise if you don't change your habits. Brain Coaching will help identify mental blocks around weight gain and set you on the right path to good habits. We address issues like:

- Why can't I lose weight? I know it is healthier for me.
- Why can't I stop smoking? I know it is affecting my breathing.
- Why can't I wear a CPAP mask? I know it will help me sleep better and my partner will thank me.

Hormones

There are many hormones involved in getting a good night's sleep. Changes in hormone levels can affect body temperature and the circadian rhythm, which are necessary for good sleep patterns. Many hormones are controlled by the sleep/wake cycle, and some are influenced by diet. The more balanced you can keep your hormones, the more likely you are to have a better sleep. You can hack your hormone levels by eating different foods, de-stressing, or taking hormone supplements. The hormones which have the most significant impact on sleep are melatonin, dopamine, serotonin and cortisol. Cortisol (stress hormone) works in close connection with melatonin (sleep hormone) – as one goes up, the other goes down. When cortisol rises, melatonin decreases, making it difficult to fall and stay asleep. When melatonin goes up, cortisol decreases, allowing you to feel less stressed and more likely to sleep easily. Too much sugar, nicotine, or caffeine at night can raise cortisol levels.

Dopamine is a neurotransmitter and is part of the 'feel-good' system in our brain. Dopamine is responsible for the 'high' we feel when we exercise, have a win in gambling, or eat chocolate. Recent research also shows that dopamine is produced in our gastrointestinal tract. Low levels of dopamine can lead to poor concentration and depression[21]. High levels of dopamine can lead to an agitated state. A high level reduces the production of melatonin.

Serotonin is a neurotransmitter that sends chemical messages to the brain. It helps regulate mood and happiness, and the sleep cycle. Low levels of serotonin can lead to depression, and depression can lead to anxiety and insomnia[22]. High serotonin levels lead to restlessness and agitation, inhibiting sleep. Most serotonin is found in the gut rather than the brain. Medications called SSRIs (Selective Serotonin Reuptake Inhibitors) are prescribed for people with depression and can improve sleep as a result. There are several types of SSRIs, and what works for one person may not work for another.

Below is a list of other hormones we naturally produce for great sleep, and a little about their roles. If you have discussed sleep issues with your GP, you may come across a name you recognise.

Adenosine – this hormone is a natural painkiller and encourages sleepiness.

Adrenalin - helps the body cope with stress, and when there is too much adrenalin, the body turns on "Fight or Flight" mode, making it difficult to fall asleep.

Adrenocorticotrophic Hormone (ACTH) – regulates cortisol levels. Levels of ACTH are usually higher in the mornings and reduce during the day, as part of a normal circadian rhythm. If the CR is out of sync, this hormone is also out, and vice versa. This may lead to higher levels of cortisol when you should be sleeping.

Aldosterone – helps maintain levels of salt and water in the body, stabilising blood pressure levels. If salt and water content increases during the night, the need to urinate will be greater. Levels of this hormone are usually higher in the mornings and decrease during the day.

Androgen – refers to the group of male hormones, although women can have smaller amounts of these hormones too. Deficiencies in these hormones can lead to sleep disruption. However, very high amounts of androgens can lead to or exacerbate sleep apnoea.

Antidiuretic Hormone (ADH) – levels of this hormone increase during sleep, thus reducing the need to wake up and pass urine. If sleep is compromised, so is the production of ADH, and a person is more likely to have the urge to urinate during the night.

Cortisol – the 'stress' hormone. Increased levels of this hormone will keep you awake at night. However, moderate levels of cortisol can help combat inflammation. Try to keep stress at moderate levels.

Dehydroepiandrosterone (DHEA) – low levels of this hormone can lead to muscle weakness. This can lead to the weakening of the pelvic floor muscles, increasing the need to pass urine during the night.

Dopamine – is a neurotransmitter rather than a hormone. Too much or too little dopamine will influence the length of sound sleep. Foods that enhance dopamine production include: bananas, almonds, dairy, meat and eggs, Vitamin B6 (found in oatmeal, brown rice, vegetables), and Vitamin C (found in citrus, kiwi fruit, pineapples, berries).

Definition: Neurotransmitters are often referred to as the body's chemical messengers. They are the molecules the nervous system uses to transmit messages between neurons, or from neurons to muscles. The brain relies on neurotransmitters to regulate many necessary functions, including - heart rate; breathing; sleep cycles; digestion; mood; concentration; appetite; muscle movement. Ref: (https://qbi.uq.edu.au/brain/brain-functions/what-are-neurotransmitters)

Ghrelin – this hormone stimulates hunger. Poor sleep leads to higher levels of ghrelin, encouraging us to overeat during the day.

Human Growth Hormone – needed for cell regeneration, growth and repair, usually released during sleep. If sleep is not happening, repair work is not occurring as well as it should.

Insulin – is a hormone secreted in the pancreas and controls the breakdown of carbohydrates, fats and proteins. It also helps the liver to store glucose and fat for energy requirements. Muscles and fat rely on insulin to uptake glucose. A drop in insulin levels, (insulin resistance), causes blood sugar levels to rise, which can eventually lead to Type 2 diabetes. If sleep is interrupted, blood sugar levels rise. The research still hasn't confirmed whether lack of sleep causes high blood sugar or whether high blood sugar causes lack of sleep. However, sleep deprivation can lead to temporary insulin resistance, most likely because of the release of stress hormones, or the increased levels of inflammatory markers such as C-reactive protein.[23]

How Does Diabetes Affect Sleep? It's estimated that one in two people (National Library of Medicine, Biotech Information) with type 2 diabetes have sleep problems because of unstable blood sugar levels and accompanying diabetes-related symptoms. High blood sugar (hyperglycaemia) and low blood sugar (hypoglycaemia) during the night can lead to insomnia and next-day fatigue. As with many chronic conditions, feelings of depression or stress about the disease itself may also keep you awake at night. When blood sugar levels are high, the kidneys overcompensate by causing you to urinate more often. During the night, these frequent trips to the bathroom lead to disrupted sleep. High blood sugar may also cause headaches and increased thirst that can interfere with falling asleep. By contrast, going too many hours without eating or taking the wrong balance of diabetes medication can also lead to low blood sugar levels at night. You may have nightmares, break out into a sweat, or feel irritated or confused when you wake up. Sleep hygiene routines should also be considered when treating patients with diabetes. (Centres for Disease Control and Prevention)

Leptin – inhibits hunger, making us feel fuller. Levels of this hormone rise during the night, so that we don't feel hungry. Poor sleep may decrease leptin levels and when levels of this hormone are low, we feel hungry, eating more to feel full.

Melatonin – too much light at nighttime reduces melatonin production, which is necessary for letting your body know it is time to sleep. Too little daytime light can also inhibit the production of melatonin. It is important to get more sunlight during the day, and less light during the evening/night. Melatonin can be found in foods like tart cherries and almonds. Many people take melatonin supplements. Some people find success with it, and others do not.

Oestrogen – when oestrogen levels drop, blood sugar rises, leading to weight gain, and increased wakefulness.

Oxytocin – also known as the 'love' hormone, oxytocin is stimulated by human touch, leaving you feeling calmer, more loving, less stressed and more likely to sleep better. Oxytocin in the bloodstream enhances parasympathetic nervous system activity – steady breathing, lower heart rate and blood pressure, and better digestion. These activities don't involve conscious thought and function while you sleep. If you are not sleeping well, then oxytocin levels may be low.

Progesterone – is one of the reproductive hormones. It promotes calm and reduces anxiety, which helps you to become sleepier.

Serotonin – when serotonin is balanced, you feel calm, and sleep is more natural. Serotonin can be increased by exercise, sunlight, improving your gut bacteria, and eating foods containing tryptophan. These include nuts, eggs, cheese, red meat, turkey, salmon, tofu, kiwi fruit and pineapple. Tryptophan[24] (an amino acid) is converted into serotonin. Serotonin can also be found in food that contains zinc, like oysters, red meat, legumes or in prescribed medications.

Testosterone – low levels of this hormone in both men and women can reduce REM sleep, leading to increased anxiety and possibly increasing the likelihood of sleep apnoea.

Please see your doctor about hormone supplements and medications.

Menopause

Sleep problems can develop during perimenopause and menopause. Many women I've worked with have listed poor sleep as a major problem during both these stages of life. They have difficulty falling asleep and/or staying asleep. One reason for sleep disruption is decreased levels of oestrogen and melatonin. Hot flushes and sweating also make sleeping very difficult. As a result, the circadian rhythm is disrupted, and the sleep/wake cycle collapses. Most menopausal women experience poor sleep, poor concentration, fatigue, and moodiness. The Australian Menopause Society (AMS) states that "insomnia is more common in women than men, and 25% of women between 50-64 years old have sleep difficulties."[25]

Officially, menopause is the period where a woman goes for a year without a menstrual cycle, and the production of oestrogen and progesterone decreases. Symptoms can include insomnia. Perimenopause is considered the stage before menopause, where a woman will experience mild symptoms of menopause, with sleeping issues among them.

You might find peri-menopausal and/or menopausal symptoms ease if you:
- Eat a healthy diet.
- Get regular exercise.
- Get enough sleep.
- Cut back on tea, coffee and other drinks with caffeine.
- Reduce stress where possible.
- Use water-based lubricants during sex.
              (Perimenopause | Healthdirect) Aust Gov. Feb 2021.

Symptoms caused by changes during perimenopause and menopause should be monitored, so that new, and possibly negative, habits, especially related to sleep routines, do not take hold and become embedded habits. Sleep problems can lead to other serious health conditions. It is important to keep on top of your sleep hygiene routine, to help mitigate symptoms during menopause, and to keep up good habits post-menopause. Having a regular sleep-wake schedule is important. As natural melatonin production declines with age, women need to spend more time outside in the daylight. Some women choose to take supplementary melatonin in a crushable form that is quickly absorbed into the system.

Other strategies could include supplementing with oestrogen tablets or Menopause Hormonal Therapy. The AMS website has some excellent fact sheets available[26]. They say that MHT has very good results improving the sleep of menopausal and post-menopausal women. They recommend that sleeping tablets be used as a last resort, mainly because of their side effects, but they also mention that anti-depressant drugs have been shown to have a sedative effect and improve sleep. Be on the alert for side effects if your doctor has recommended this course of action.

Brain Coaching helps encourage peri-menopausal-through-to-post-menopausal women to be mindful of their habits and establish better mental and physical behaviours.

Sexual Intercourse and Sleep

"Sex, like most aspects of our health, all starts with sleep."
(Chris Brantner, SleepZoo.com)

Some say that your bed should be reserved for only two activities – sleep and sex. Your bed is not for working, or movies, or eating because, when you think about it, if you are doing these things, you are not sleeping or paying attention to your partner!

Many trials have been conducted on issues related to sex and its subsequent effect on sleep[27] which show a bidirectional effect – less sleep leads to less sex, and less sex leads to less sleep.

So, what is actually going on here? And does it mean that the opposite is true? More sex equals more sleep?.

The obvious reason for less sleep leading to less sex is a person feeling too tired or having less libido to engage in sex. Less sex can factor into keeping you awake - you feel frustrated, you feel neglected, you feel resentment, you feel insecure and negative thoughts arise: *Aren't I attractive enough?*

How about turning this around? Have more sex and see if your sleep improves. During sex, the hormone oxytocin is released. This is also called the 'love' hormone. It is activated through the caring touch in humans – one of the 'feel-good' hormones, and it can relieve stress. Other feel-good hormones like endorphins, oestrogen, prolactin, and dopamine can also be released after having satisfying sexual intercourse. Of course, everyone is different; some will feel too stimulated to sleep, and others will be more relaxed. Surveys have been conducted that say around 60% of respondents sleep better after satisfying sex[28]. Physical and emotional closeness is just as important as actual sexual intercourse in promoting feel-good hormones.

Everyday stress can lead to sleep disruption, anxiety and depression. When stressed, the brain can suppress sex hormones, like testosterone and oestrogen, which can lead to subsequent sexual dysfunction in both males and females. If this is the case for you or someone you know, psychotherapy or Brain Coaching can help.

As your Brain Coach, I help identify the underlying cause of sleep problems and/or sexual dysfunction. Then, together, we will formulate strategies to overcome these issues that suit your individual lifestyle and relationship.

Some strategies may include regular mild exercise. This can help lower cortisol levels, relax the body, and improve sex drive. Reducing alcohol intake and cigarette smoking can also improve libido.

As researchers Lastella et al., said in their paper - *"Sexual intercourse as a possible alternative or addition to other intervention strategies for insomnia*[28] — intriguing possibility, hey?

BUT!!! – I hear you say …

"I feel unattractive."

That is a matter of opinion, of course. Brain Coaching helps you feel better about yourself and creates new thought patterns about what exactly is 'attractiveness.'

"I am too tired."

We can work together on how to overcome feelings of exhaustion.

"I don't have time."

I know of one couple who made a concerted effort to have sex every day, no matter how quick it was, even if they were tired (they also had young children). The outcome was that they were always thinking of the other person, had increased oxytocin, and felt more loved. Amazing! We can do anything if we make a concerted effort and put our minds to it!

Brain Coaching can help modify your mindset and make you feel more confident and committed.

Chapter summary

Keeping a sleep diary can help you identify patterns in your daily life. You can monitor what works and what doesn't work for you. Record your daily exercise, when and at what intensity; record what you consume – meals, coffee, alcohol, tablets, etc. Record your nightly routine. You should be able to notice patterns after four weeks. I have devised a comprehensive sleep diary. It considers all the factors in your daily life that can impact your sleep.

See Appendix B for your blank Sleep Diary and visit my website if you need more. This Diary is quite comprehensive and shows how many factors are in your life that can impact on sleep.

There are many areas related to sleep that you can influence on your own. Which of these could you be focusing on?

- ☐ Circadian Rhythm – adequate daylight, nightly routines.
- ☐ Diet and supporting your Gut/Brain connection – what and when to eat.
- ☐ Vagus nerve – stimulating this nerve to keep your systems in balance.
- ☐ Exercise – how much and when you move impacts different systems in the body.
- ☐ Hydration – importance of balancing fluid intake, and the impacts of under or overhydration.
- ☐ Obesity – weight gain affects your body, breathing and sleep.
- ☐ Hormones –by relieving stress, making food choices or using supplements or see your doctor for more serious hormone-related issues.
- ☐ Menopause – changes in hormone levels will result in sweating, hot flushes and disrupted sleep.
- ☐ Sexual intercourse - satisfying activities can lead to better sleep, and better sleep could lead to more sex. Could there be more sex in your future?
- ☐ Stress reduction techniques – to prepare your mind for bed.

How can Brain Coaching help address the physiological issues discussed above?

Brain Coaching identifies triggers causing your sleep issues and works to overcome any emotional blocks caused by those triggers. You know the lifestyle changes you need to make to improve your sleep, so let's look at that together. Having support makes starting new changes so much easier. Your success is important to me. Here are some questions I can help you answer:

- Do I just feel too tired?
- Do I feel I'm just not worth the effort?
- Is it all too hard? "I'll just put up with less sleep."
- Do I need to address my weight to help me breathe better when I'm sleeping?
- Do I need to optimise my exercise times?
- Do I need to reduce stress?
- Would I like help to improve my sex life?
- Do I need to stop procrastinating and go to bed at a reasonable hour?
- Do I need motivation to stop the late-night snacking?
- Do I need help to retrain my brain and my bladder so that the need to urinate is not waking me up?

Addressing physiological issues and improving your sleep by implementing minor tweaks, or body-hacks, could ease health problems before they become more serious. If being overweight is causing breathing problems and sleep apnoea, addressing this could also avoid heart problems. If stress is leading to digestive disorders, managing the stress will avoid medical intervention and improve sleep.

Brain Coaching unlocks your blocks, renews your motivation, and removes that sense of helplessness. Yes, you are worth the effort! Brain Coaching will help eliminate procrastination, encourage commitment, and build the consistency to achieve your goals.

Imagine how amazing you will feel when you create new habits and improve your sleep!

If you could only have one car for life, how would you look after it?

*"Knowing it had to last a lifetime, what would I do with it? I would read the manual about five times. I would always keep it garaged. If there were the least little dent or scratch, I'd have it fixed right away because I wouldn't want it rusting. I would baby that car because it would have to last a lifetime. That's exactly the position you are in concerning your mind and body. You only get one mind and one body. And it's got to last a lifetime. Now, it's very easy to let them ride for many years. But if you don't take care of that mind and that body, you'll be a wreck forty years later, just like the car would be. It's what you do right now, today, that determines how your mind and body will operate ten, twenty, and thirty years from now." – **Warren Buffett.**

CHAPTER 6

Medical Issues
that Can Affect Sleep

"There is more refreshment and stimulation in a nap, even of the briefest, than in all the alcohol ever distilled."
Edward Lucas, British Writer

Sleep is restorative. While we sleep, systems in the body important for good health repair and regroup, readying us to fight infections, heart disease, cancer, inflammatory diseases and depression[1]. Have you already been diagnosed with a medical condition? Chances are that your medical condition is affecting how well you sleep and not sleeping well, may exacerbate your physical symptoms.

Alternatively, your sleep problems could be caused by a medical condition that hasn't yet been diagnosed. Pain is an obvious reason sleep might be interrupted, whereas a thyroid problem is not as obvious, and can often take time to diagnose. Some people put up with these conditions thinking, *"Oh, it is just the way I am," or "It's just because I can't sleep".*

Only later do they discover a medical condition is the cause of sleep issues. Please don't ignore symptoms – your health and your sleep depend on a correct diagnosis. If you are unsure whether you have a medical issue, a visit to your doctor will eliminate any guesswork. It is vital to resolve possible medical reasons for your insomnia before you go down the path of alternative solutions. There are many medical conditions that can disrupt sleep patterns. Our goal is to prevent disturbed sleep from becoming a habit that the body and brain become used to. We want to prevent disturbed sleep from progressing to chronic insomnia, which can then lead to further issues.

Is it the medical problem that causes sleep disruption or sleep disruption which leads to a medical condition?

Either scenario could mask what is really happening. Again, getting all possible medical reasons checked out by your doctor is very important. Once you have a suspected medical condition sorted but still have trouble sleeping, Brain Coaching can help you get back on track with a healthier sleep routine.

In the following paragraphs, I present information on medical conditions that could be affecting your sleep. You will also find helpful tips that may restore a better sleep pattern.

If you have, or suspect you have, any of these conditions, please seek medical advice first. Your sleep and your health depend on a correct diagnosis.

Poor Circulation

Have you ever had trouble going to sleep or waking up during the night because your hands or feet are too hot or too cold? A functioning circulation system ensures that nutrients, blood and oxygen are transported effectively and with a regular flow around the body. It also means that toxins and waste products are transported away and excreted from the body.

Poor circulation can affect our sleep and our cardiovascular health. Poor circulation can also lead to sleep apnoea, obesity and atherosclerosis (clogging of the arteries).

Sleep and circulation share a bidirectional relationship. A good night's sleep improves circulation and, if circulation improves, so does your sleep. The same can be said for the opposite – poor sleep can lead to circulation problems, and poor circulation can lead to disrupted sleep. It is important to maintain a healthy circulatory system to prevent issues that will keep you awake.

Symptoms of poor circulation can include: swelling of feet (oedema), discoloured, cold/numb hands and feet, or tingling or cramps in the extremities. Lack of oxygen circulating in our bloodstream can lead to: fatigue, poor memory, dizziness, dry skin, slow healing of wounds, or shortness of breath.

It's important to find out the reason for poor circulation if you have any of these symptoms. Please see your doctor if you are experiencing symptoms of poor circulation.

Some treatments that aid circulation include:

- Putting a pillow under your feet at night so the feet are elevated.
- Exercising during the day and opting for gentle feet and leg exercises in the evening.
- Healthy diet, antioxidant-rich food and drinks, adequate water.
- Feet and leg massages and/or stretching.
- Compression stockings.
- Quit smoking.
- Reduce alcohol consumption.
- Reduce stress.

Hot or Cold Feet

Poor circulation can lead to hot or cold feet. Having hot, throbbing feet at night can be uncomfortable and keep you awake. People with diabetes, or those who consume too much alcohol, can experience hot feet. A hot burning sensation in the feet can also indicate a vitamin deficiency. It is important to get a medical diagnosis for the actual cause of hot or cold feet to implement the correct treatment. Natural remedies might help: supplements like antioxidants, amino acids, turmeric, evening primrose oil and vitamins have all been recommended. Wearing comfortable shoes or compression socks during the day, having foot baths with magnesium salts, or activities to cool the feet before bed are helpful. First, check with your medical practitioner.

Cold feet can keep you awake as they take time to warm up. A remedy could be as simple as wearing warm socks to bed. Nerve stimulation therapies or acupuncture may also be helpful in some cases.

Hot or cold feet and limbs can be more than just a nuisance, particularly if it disturbs your sleep. We want to prevent sleep disturbance from becoming a habit. It is important to discover the underlying cause first, treat it, then work on getting your sleep back in to a normal rhythm.

Sleep Apnoea

Sleep Apnoea is a medical condition that is more than just a snoring problem, and can be dangerous to your health if not treated. Not only does it result in interrupted sleep, but sleep apnoea can lead to heart problems and high blood pressure.

Symptoms of sleep apnoea include: noisy snoring/breathing/gasping during sleep, dry throat when waking, daytime sluggishness, headaches when waking, poor concentration and memory, moodiness and irritability. These symptoms could indicate that less oxygen is travelling to the brain.

Causes of Sleep Apnoea include: obesity, small airways, smoking and high blood pressure.

A meta-analysis of five different research studies completed in 2014[2] found that exercise training reduced the severity of sleep breathing disorders by up to 30% in patients. The participants didn't even need to lose weight for the exercise to influence their breathing while they were asleep. Results were noticed after four weeks. However, the exercise training must be sustained to impact overall health. This exercise regime also positively impacted daytime drowsiness, depressive episodes, fatigue, and energy levels. Some researchers found that exercise could have facilitated fluid draining from the legs. They recommended people should at least try for a less sedentary lifestyle, even if they aren't capable of vigorous exercise.

It's easy to fall into a cycle of not exercising because you are tired. As a result of not exercising, your symptoms persist or worsen. Just a small effort can deliver significant rewards.

Other respiratory problems that impact sleep:

- Shallow or restricted breathing as a result of panic/anxiety.
- Respiratory infections.
- Chronic Obstructive Pulmonary Disease (COPD).
- Nasal Congestion.
- Deviated Septum.
- Restricted breathing due to acid reflux.
- Hypoventilation is when carbon dioxide is retained in the body due to shallow breathing.

Tips for improving breathing problems:

- Regular exercise.
- Weight loss.
- Deep breathing, to reduce stress and oxygenate the blood.
- Sleep with head slightly raised to reduce reflux impediments.
- Use CPAP, ASV or Jaw (Mandibula) Splints if recommended.

A CPAP (Continuous Positive Airways Pressure) is a device that pumps purified air into your nose and mouth. It involves wearing a fitted mask while you are sleeping. It keeps the airways open by sending a steady flow of oxygen into the nose and mouth, and helps you breathe normally. It also helps to stop the tongue from lolling back into the throat and blocking the airway. When breathing is enabled and back to normal, waking up to breathe and gasping for air are eliminated. When fitted properly, a person becomes used to wearing the CPAP mask, and many find it improves their sleep, reporting subsequent improvements in their daily lives. They feel more alert; relationships improve, mood improves, blood pressure reduces, and the risk of depression and heart problems is lowered. There can be limited drawbacks: dry mouth and throat, skin irritation from the mask, or feeling anxious about wearing a mask. Some people are reluctant to wear the mask and miss out on reaping the benefits.

Adaptive servo-ventilation (ASV) machines monitor a person's breathing while they sleep and deliver customised air pressure to stabilize breathing. The main difference between ASV and CPAP machines is that ASV machines deliver air pressure dynamically, adjusting according to the person's breathing patterns. In contrast, CPAP machines deliver a set level of air pressure throughout the night. Each device has specific benefits depending on the cause of sleep apnoea. (National Library of Medicine, Biotech Information USA.)

CASE STUDIES

Drew, a young man in his thirties with sleep apnoea, who used to be overweight, had terrible sleeping patterns, and had depression. He said that he used to feel like a zombie walking around during the day.

Drew has been using an ASV machine (alternative to the CPAP machine) successfully for fourteen years and felt fantastic right from the start. He now averages about 8hrs sleep per night. Drew also said that his temperament has improved. He strongly recommends the use of this Positive Airways machine to people with snoring problems. Some people say that the ASV machine is less claustrophobic than the CPAP, (which has put some people off from wearing them).

Anthony, a Jaw Splint Recipient – *"For years I have been feeling sluggish and tired in the afternoons, so much so that I become unproductive and reliant on coffee to keep me going!*

I had assumed that everyone felt that way, though I started to realise that isn't true… most people can function well for an entire day without needing a nap (certainly people in their 30's!).

I finally spoke to a 'Snore' specialist who diagnosed me with mild sleep apnoea. Turns out my snoring is not only annoying to my wife, but is a symptom of my tongue blocking my airway when I lie on my back. When this happens, I can't breathe, so I wake up slightly, which leads to poor and inconsistent sleep. The solution? Something called a mandibula splint…

Basically, it's a double mouthguard that holds my bottom jaw forward (painlessly) and prevents my tongue from blocking my throat, allowing me to breathe without strain, leading to deeper, consistent sleep throughout the night.

The result was instant - I am no longer snoring, I can work effectively throughout the day, and I wake up actually feeling refreshed in the morning. I didn't think anything could have been done without surgery, but this was a fantastic investment in my health that I can't recommend enough."

Thyroid Dysregulation

Thyroxine is a hormone released by the thyroid gland. Thyroxine is necessary for the proper function of most organs and is vital to many processes, such as breathing, heart rate, digestion, and body temperature. Under or over-production of thyroxine can lead to health problems, including anxiety and insomnia. Iodine intake plays a key part in thyroid function or dysfunction. The thyroid gland uses iodine to produce thyroxine, so too little or too much iodine in your diet may contribute to thyroid issues.

Thyroid problems have been linked to sleep problems. Hyperthyroidism (overactive thyroid) can disrupt sleep because metabolism increases. Your system becomes overstimulated, leading to irritable moods, muscle weakness, and constant tiredness. Hyperactive thyroid may also cause night sweats and the urge to frequently urinate, which disrupts sleep.

People with hypothyroidism (underactive thyroid), often have trouble sleeping because they feel cold at night and can experience joint or muscle pain that disrupts sleep. An underactive thyroid has been linked to taking longer to fall asleep and experiencing shorter sleep durations. *"Untreated hypothyroidism can be mistaken for sleep-related hypoventilation, or excessively slow or shallow breathing that occurs primarily during sleep"*[3].

Hypothyroidism: Also known as Hashimoto's disease, develops when the thyroid gland is underactive, usually caused by low iodine levels or the body's inability to produce thyroid hormones necessary for growth and development (an autoimmune deficiency). Insomnia is one symptom. This condition affects about 1 in 20 people, mainly women. Treatment includes increasing iodine intake, or thyroid hormone medication[4].

Hyperthyroidism: Also known as Grave's disease, is caused by an overactive thyroid gland and affects about 1 in 100 people. The thyroid produces an excessive amount of hormone, and metabolism speeds up. Treatment includes medications to lower the thyroid hormone levels[5].

Thyroid problems and sleep problems can be bidirectional, an over or underactive thyroid can lead to disrupted sleep, and continually disrupted sleep can lead to thyroid imbalances. Good quality sleep supports a healthy immune system, and people with a weakened immune system are at higher risk of developing an illness like thyroid dysfunction. It is important to have your thyroid levels checked as thyroid issues can cause health problems, which you may put down to just sleep problems. Or the opposite could be true, your sleep problems could mask a thyroid problem.

Tips on how to deal with hyperthyroidism:

- Maintain healthy iodine levels (avoid foods high in iodine).
- Include selenium-rich foods.
- Increase probiotics.
- Cut back on sugar intake.
- Exercise regularly.
- Manage stress.
- Pharmaceuticals.
- Surgery to remove thyroid gland.

Tips on dealing with hypothyroidism:

- Manage stress and depression.
- Exercise regularly.

- Include enough iodine in the diet (150mg/day – usually half a teaspoon of iodised salt).
- Include tyrosine, (amino acid supplement), or it can be found in seaweed, turkey, eggs.
- Include vitamin D – found in fatty fish, eggs or yoghurt.
- Include antioxidants – found in berries, nuts, green vegetables.
- Include selenium – found in nuts, seeds, eggs, seafood, or a supplement of 200mg/day.
- Include vitamin B12 – found in poultry, fish, meat, or a vegan supplement.
- Avoid foods with excess sodium, soy products, antacids.
- Thyroid medications.

Pain

It is very difficult to get a good night's sleep if you are suffering from pain, whether it is acute pain (usually short term) or chronic pain (long term). Pain is the body's way of sending messages to the brain, via our nervous system, letting it know that something is wrong, and we need to do something about it. Sometimes pain can seem more severe or noticeable when we finally go to bed and can rest. Anxiety, whether from lack of sleep, or the anxiety causing lack of sleep, can make people feel more sensitive to pain. They may even have a heightened sense of expectancy, i.e., *"I'm in for a bad night, bet I can't sleep because the pain will come back,"* and a sleeplessness/pain cycle begins.

Waking up exhausted makes us less likely to make healthy lifestyle choices the next day, compounding, and possibly leading to further symptoms, including depression. There have been studies conducted in America which found that about 40% of people with chronic pain also have depression.[6] Distress caused by pain can also lead to sleeplessness. Tiredness throughout the day, along with having to deal with pain, can also lead to feeling unsociable and not wanting to exercise, impacting our quality of sleep. This can lead to a pain-depression cycle, when all you can think about is the pain you are in and how tired you are. When considering this interaction, it is sometimes advisable to treat both the pain symptoms and the depression symptoms at the same time, with either pharmaceuticals, exercise and/or behaviour therapy to retrain your brain.

Medications like opioids are not necessarily the answer. They have their own set of side-effects and repercussions. Some opioids used as pain medication can cause breathing problems while sleeping, and the possibility of reliance, addiction and reduced efficacy of the medication.

Suggestions for drug-free pain treatment:

- Sleeping positions can relieve pain. If your pain is caused by pressure points - use a pillow between the legs when you sleep on your side.
- If you have back pain, then sleeping with lumbar support may relieve pain.
- Pain or discomfort from indigestion may be relieved by sleeping with two pillows in an elevated position.
- Relaxation exercises are widely recommended for people with pain.
- Massage for pain relief.
- Meditation, mindfulness and distraction are also worthwhile practising to take your mind off the pain and help to promote sleep.

Pain is real. However, there have been many research trials that show how, in some instances, pain can be managed by retraining the brain. In 2021, researchers at Helsinki University[7] ran a study on post-operative patients who had pain after an operation. They found that these patients, who had reported severe pain and insomnia, could improve their sleep quality and pain levels by reducing their tendency to expect pain and catastrophise about their condition. When patients think *"I'm never going to get better*, or *the pain will be so bad, I'll never sleep again"*. Their anxiety increases, sleep is jeopardised, and post-operative recovery takes longer. Researchers found that brain re-training could help lower their catastrophising, reduce stress, improve their sleep, and lower pain intensity.

Pain and sleep can share a bidirectional relationship – one can influence the other. Brain Coaching helps people with chronic pain come to terms with their injury, or the reason for the pain, and develop new thought patterns and diversions. Brain Coaching helps to motivate people living with pain to keep making the right decisions for their health. The result of Brain Coaching intervention will be better sleep and reduced sensitivity to pain. When re-training the brain using mindfulness and distraction techniques, we establish positive thought patterns and routines to replace negative habits. Getting on top of your sleep issues will help with the pain, and solving your pain issues will bring you better sleep. This may seem obvious but many people are still suffering. Are you ready to take control of your pain?

CASE STUDY

Pete, a man in his forties with chronic lower back pain, had trouble sleeping, and was very grumpy and argumentative with those around him. He also had a very stressful life – pressure at work, a young family, a mortgage, and his marriage was suffering. During Brain Coaching, we discovered that his stress accentuated his pain. Once we worked out the exact reason for the stress, and resolved that issue, then he could work on some strategies to mitigate the intensity of the pain. Prior to Brain Coaching, it was almost like his brain was expecting the pain. That is, his senses were heightened, so that he actually felt the pain even when the injury was no longer there. He had seen doctors for x-rays and MRIs, and they said there was no sign of injury there. The doctors diagnosed that his back had recovered and suggested that he seek psychological or behavioural therapy. The original damage had been and gone. So why was he still feeling this excruciating pain? His brain had become over-sensitised to expect it. After Brain Coaching and a few weeks of reinforcing new thinking patterns, the pain had gone away. He said he felt like a new man, and was sleeping much better as a result. His relationships improved, too.

Immune System and Autoimmune Diseases

The primary causes or risk factors for various autoimmune diseases are thought to be genetic or lifestyle-related. Genetically, it is possible to inherit a predisposition for an autoimmune disease, however, it isn't guaranteed that you will develop this disease. Environmental factors that can trigger autoimmune disease include: toxins that we live and work with, stress, infections, diet, or a compromised gut biome. Experiencing disrupted sleep as a result of an autoimmune diagnosis, or other factors, makes it harder for your body to combat autoimmune disease.

Food choices can significantly impact our sleep pattern and our immune system, often with a reciprocal effect. Changes in our lifestyle and diet can improve our ability to fight infections and reduce the incidence and/or severity of inflammatory autoimmune diseases. Plant-based diets have been shown to improve our gut bacteria and our sleep. Reducing the fat, sugar and gluten in our daily intake has been shown to improve our immune system[8].

Chronic tiredness during the day can be an early indicator of various autoimmune diseases[9]. Autoimmune diseases can affect sleep because of the pain, discomfort, symptoms, and depression these various diseases bring.

All systems in the body are linked, and sleep underpins all the body's functions. Sleep boosts the immune system. Current medical thinking suggests that when the immune system is weakened, it attacks the body's own tissue, resulting in an autoimmune disease.

A well-functioning immune system is vital for the body to fight off infections and identify self-tissue and non-self-tissue (foreign bodies, toxins). When you are sleeping, the brain goes through a series of electromagnetic currents, or waves. During deep sleep, the most restful stage of sleep, muscles are relaxed. This is when your immune system is boosted and the body can fight the infection more effectively. The cortisol or stress hormones should be at their lowest levels in this stage of sleep, but if you are sleep-deprived, cortisol levels rise, leading to a stress response where adrenalin is released into your system, which then leads to suppression of the immune system and inflammation occurs.

In his research paper[12], Krueger (2016) explains how the immune system affects sleep in various ways. He describes how infections can cause a number of responses, including a lack of energy and tiredness. This could be why people who are sick need more time sleeping, to recover. Sleep structure changes during infection, altering how much time is spent in certain sleep stages. Usually, people spend more time in stage three non-rapid eye movement (NREM) sleep or deep sleep during an infection. This is the sleep stage where bodily processes slow right down, making it more likely for the body's immune system to utilise energy to fight the infection. Your body needs good quality sleep to fight infectious diseases.

Even though you feel you are getting enough sleep, the quality of that sleep is important to enhance your immune system. Studies have shown that people who sleep better respond better to vaccinations. Poor sleepers are often more prone to infections. Poor sleep can mean the flight-or-fight response is heightened while the body is supposed to be resting. This fight-or-flight response increases the production of stress hormones and reduces the immune response, which can lead to the immune system having a lower response rate to vaccinations. The vaccination is not as efficient in people who have poor sleep[10].

Lack of sleep weakens our immune system, making us prone to infections and illnesses, and slows down recovery. Sleep improves t-cell function. T-cells are a type of immune cell. T-cells detect foreign pathogens and release cytokines (proteins) to attack pathogens. Cortisol (the stress hormone) decreases the efficiency of T-cells in killing pathogens and warding off disease[11].

In the short-term, lack of sleep can make us prone to infections like cold or flu. Lack of sleep in the long-term can cause low-level systemic inflammation in the body, which may lead to an increased risk of diabetes, cardiovascular and neurodegenerative diseases, and other autoimmune diseases and depression.[11] Part of dealing with or preventing autoimmune diseases is learning how to deal with stress and build mental and physical resilience. Brain Coaching can help. Self-care is so important. When we place more value on taking care of ourselves and our health, we can avoid succumbing to an ongoing cycle of stress, sleeplessness, and disease. Behavioural changes that improve sleep can reduce the impact of any cycle of illness and loss of sleep, possibly without the need for drugs. See the Good Habits guide in the Appendix A.

The most common autoimmune diseases include: diabetes; rheumatoid arthritis; psoriasis; multiple sclerosis; lupus; inflammatory bowel disease (IBD including Crohn's & ulcerative colitis); Addison's disease; hyperthyroidism; vasculitis; coeliac's disease; fibromyalgia; chronic fatigue syndrome, adrenal fatigue, and more. *(See Appendix F for a comprehensive list of AI diseases)*

As with any serious health conditions, it is extremely important to consult with your medical practitioner first, to identify and treat and/or rule out likely causes of the ailments.

Narcolepsy

Narcolepsy is a chronic neurological disorder that affects the brain's ability to control sleep-wake cycles, and causes spells of REM sleep, the state where you dream, during the day. These 'fits' of inappropriate sleep can last from a few seconds to thirty minutes. People with narcolepsy may feel rested immediately after waking in the morning, but then feel very sleepy throughout the day. Many individuals with narcolepsy also experience interrupted sleep during the night.[13]

The most common symptom of narcolepsy is falling asleep at the drop of a hat, during the day, at inappropriate times. Some people even fall asleep during pleasurable activities, meetings, or driving. It is the second most common cause of **excessive daytime sleepiness (EDS)** after sleep apnoea. Statistics from the Australian Brain Foundation on the number of people who have been diagnosed with narcolepsy indicate that it occurs in about one per thousand people in European countries, Japan and the United States.[12] Narcolepsy can go undiagnosed for years as many people simply think they are tired from lack of sleep. Other forms of narcolepsy include:

- **Cataplexy** - a "sudden episode of muscle weakness triggered by heightened emotions." (sleepfoundation.org).
- **Sleep paralysis** – where a person suddenly finds themselves unable to move for a few minutes, even though they are fully conscious.
- **Hypnagogic hallucinations** – dream-like hallucinations while about to fall asleep.

Not everyone with a type of narcolepsy experiences all the above conditions. The development and severity of the above symptoms will vary with each person. It is important to get a correct diagnosis, which usually includes a sleep latency test measuring the time it takes to get to sleep. Testing also checks for other possible reasons for the sleep disorder. People who suffer from narcolepsy usually fall asleep within five minutes of the test beginning, and they move into REM sleep quickly, compared to normal sleepers.

Narcolepsy can be difficult to diagnose. It is vital to get a correct diagnosis for three reasons:

- Narcolepsy must be managed correctly.
- These symptoms may mask the diagnosis of something else.
- Narcolepsy puts the sufferer in potential danger, e.g., when in the car or in the bath.

At this stage, researchers say there is no cure, but Narcolepsy can be managed by medication or behavioural intervention. Behavioural intervention includes – avoiding highly emotional situations (although it is difficult to anticipate these), scheduling daytime naps (instead of relying on random naps) and establishing a regular night-time routine.

Brain Coaching can help with behavioural interventions.

Restless Leg Syndrome (RLS)

RLS, also known as Willis-Ekbom Disease, occurs in about 5-15% of the population and in most cases, the cause is unknown [14]. It can be related to obesity, or low iron or magnesium levels. RLS disrupts your sleep, and your partner's sleep. Symptoms include feelings of itchy, crawling, prickling skin, and/or twitching spasmodic muscle movement, particularly of the legs. RLS is related to dopamine (the feel-good hormone) receptors in the brain, and the amount of oxygen getting to the brain. Snoring or sleep apnoea reduces the level of oxygen in the brain while sleeping, and there is a recognised connection between sleep apnoea and RLS. Restless Leg Syndrome prevalence in patients with Sleep Apnoea Syndrome varies between 7 and 36%, which is higher than in the general population.[15]

Treatment includes: iron supplements; avoiding caffeine, alcohol, and cigarettes; losing weight; taking magnesium supplements; or pharmaceuticals. Some pharmaceuticals used to treat RLS can have detrimental effects on a person's emotional wellbeing or lifestyle. Labels warn about the potential loss of inhibitions. Short-term side effects of recommended medications are usually mild, including nausea, light-headedness and fatigue. Long-term use can cause impulse control disorders, such as compulsive gambling, daytime sleepiness or addiction.[16]

"Caution about medications. Sometimes dopamine medications that have worked for a while to relieve your RLS become ineffective. Some medications may worsen symptoms of RLS"[16].

If you have tried medical and behavioural solutions and still suffer from RLS, retraining your brain will help. Pharmaceuticals can have unwanted side effects, and exploring other options may be worthwhile. Brain Coaching reveals whether emotional triggers are the reason for RLS, identifies triggers that may have potentially caused this condition, and addresses the way your brain perceives these to enable you to get better sleep.

Lack of Essential Nutrients

Essential vitamins and minerals are necessary for good health, and good sleep. A lack of essential nutrients can lead to adverse medical conditions, if not addressed. Supplements are a popular way to boost levels of certain vitamins and minerals. Nutritional deficiency is linked to insomnia and may be alleviated by taking relevant supplements or eating a wide variety of whole foods. Whole foods are foods in/or close to their natural state, or minimally processed.

A well-known essential mineral linked to tiredness is iron. Our bodies can go into a state of anaemia when iron levels are low. Most of us know that a lack of iron can cause us to feel tired and lethargic during the day, but a lack of iron can also cause disrupted sleep during the night.

Iron deficiency is also associated with restless leg syndrome, which causes wakefulness at night. Iron deficiency can also result in increased anxiety, and symptoms can be implicated in other disorders. It is important to have a correct diagnosis of iron deficiency to ensure appropriate treatment.

A note of caution: self-dosing with too much iron could damage your liver. It is very important to consult your doctor, who will conduct blood tests to ascertain your iron levels.

In 2019, a team of researchers at British Columbia University[17] conducted a major scoping review of 93 research trials worldwide that dealt with iron deficiency and sleep disorders in children and older adults. Their results showed an *"over-whelming positive correlation"* between iron levels and the amount of sleep. The studies also found that iron supplements helped in most cases, including children with low iron levels.

Other minerals and nutrients that are essential for good sleep include: Vitamins A, B, C, D, E, calcium, magnesium, and potassium, as well as some micronutrients. [18]

Table: List of essential vitamins and minerals that can aid sleep[19]

Element	Needed for	Source
Iron	production of neurotransmitters like dopamine, serotonin, noradrenaline	red meat, fish, eggs, nuts, dried fruit, dark green leafy vegetables
Magnesium	reducing stress and blood pressure, boosting metabolism, and relaxing nerves and muscles	nuts, spinach, black beans, soy, whole wheat bread, avocado, and potatoes.
Tryptophan	production of melatonin that helps induce and maintain sleep, REM sleep phase	dairy, eggs, green vegetables, sardines and soybeans
Vitamin B12	increasing the production of melatonin, important for regulating sleep-wake cycles	beef, fish, eggs, chicken, and dairy products

Element	Needed for	Source
Vitamin B6	production of serotonin and melatonin, helps metabolise protein	chickpeas, tuna, chicken, potatoes, turkey, and bananas
Vitamin C	antioxidant properties, may help increase sleep duration, reduce sleep disturbances, relieve movement disorders, and may decrease the dangerous effects of sleep apnoea	citrus fruit, red and green peppers, berries, broccoli, spinach
Vitamin D	production of melatonin and helps the absorption of calcium	sunshine, mushrooms
Omega 3 Fatty Acid	improving sleep quality and ability to fall asleep more quickly	fatty fish, canola oil, flaxseed, chia seeds, and walnuts
Potassium	preventing muscle cramps, which can disrupt sleep	dried apricots, lentils, raisins, potatoes, kidney beans, soy, and bananas
Vitamin E	antioxidant properties	nuts, seeds, spinach, broccoli, tomatoes
Vitamin A	regulating the circadian rhythm	leafy green vegetables, orange and yellow vegetables, tomato products, fruits, and some vegetable oils

Using diet and nutrition to improve sleep can be a less expensive, less intrusive, and more convenient strategy than using pharmaceuticals to enhance sleep and subsequently overall health.

Nocturia

Nocturia is the need to urinate at night. Many people state that having to urinate during the night is the main reason their sleep is broken and they can't get back to sleep. The good news is, unless there is a medical reason for needing to void during the night, you can retrain your brain and your bladder. Physiologically, it is normal to go all night without needing to go to the toilet.

Medical reasons for needing to urinate during the night can include[20]:

- Polyuria – passing a high volume of urine, possibly caused by high fluid intake; diabetes; or high blood sugar.
- Nocturnal urinary frequency – needing to pass small amounts often during the night, possibly caused by habit; bladder obstructions; urinary tract infection; or enlarged prostate.
- Nocturnal polyuria – passing high volume only at night-time, possibly caused by heart problems; oedema; sleep apnoea; diuretic drugs; high sodium diet; or too much caffeine or alcohol.

Interventions can include:

- Keeping a urination diary to help identify patterns.
- Restrict fluids, especially in the evenings.
- Elevate the legs in bed.
- Wear compression stockings.
- Therapy to re-train your brain and your bladder.

Once sleep is interrupted consistently, wakefulness can become a habit, leading to problems related to health, relationships, and productivity.

CASE STUDY

Chris is the manager of a busy retail outlet, overseeing forty staff, as well as dealing with customers, and juggling a young family. Life was pretty stressful. Chris had trouble sleeping and went to the toilet five times a night. His sleep was very disrupted, and he had to cope with family and work issues the next day. His anxiety was at a very high level. During Brain Coaching, we identified why he felt the need to get up so often to urinate during the night. It wasn't a physical or medical problem, it was an emotional issue, and his brain and his bladder had got into the habit of 'needing' to empty often. We helped resolve that issue and came up with some strategies to assist sleep. Chris now sleeps through the night, is a lot calmer at work, and handles life's stresses more relaxed and less emotionally. Chris is much more productive, too. He is so relieved and proud of himself.

In this case we concentrated on the logic of the situation – there was no physical or medical need to get up so often during the night. Chris was able to retrain his brain and his bladder!

Chapter summary

Sleep deprivation is implicated in most chronic health disorders and living with a medical condition can lead to new or further sleep complications. Sleep complications can increase our vulnerability to a medical condition. Research trials have identified that compromised sleep patterns leaves likely, or potential sufferers with repressed immune systems. Treatments can be targeted and implemented before disease and/or other negative consequences of poor sleep can take effect.

The following list summarises symptoms that could potentially be the cause of medically related sleep problems:

☐ Hot or cold hands and feet, poor circulation, tingling.
☐ Breathing problems: snoring, apnoea, irregular breathing, nasal congestion, reflux, shallow breathing (hypoventilation).
☐ Night-sweats – menopause, or hyperthyroidism (over-active metabolism).
☐ Pain, or pressure points, anywhere in the body - acute (short term), chronic (long term), temporary or dull aches.
☐ Gut problems – bloating, tightness, constipation, indigestion, reflux.
☐ Autoimmune diseases – various symptoms.
☐ Depression.
☐ Infection.
☐ Falling asleep at inappropriate times.
☐ Restless legs, especially when sitting or lying down.
☐ Urinating often during the night.
☐ Extreme daytime fatigue.

If you have any of the above symptoms, please seek medical advice to resolve the issue before it becomes chronic, disrupting your sleep consistently and leading to further problems.

It's important to properly diagnose and treat any medical condition to improve health and eliminate or minimise further sleep disruption.

Many research trials have been conducted on sleep architecture and its impacts, and results have shown benefits from various pharmaceuticals and behavioural treatments, with behavioural therapies providing significant benefits at less cost. Behavioural treatments are generally more successful, efficient, and cheaper than other types of treatment. Irwin in 2022 found that behavioural therapies like Cognitive Behavioural Therapy (CBT), yoga, and meditation positively affected the sleep/stress cycle[21].

Brain Coaching is a form of CBT, however Brain Coaching goes further by first identifying the root cause of the insomnia and resolves that issue, before introducing relevant and appropriate behavioural strategies. When you don't recognise the original cause of sleeplessness, it's almost impossible to resolve the issue; the problem will continue to crop up, and chronic insomnia may result.

BUT!!! - I hear you say …

"I've got a diagnosis and I can't sleep … "

Together we can work on following and maximising medical advice. You don't have to take this journey alone.

"I am too busy to look into this problem, or to see a doctor - it's only minor."

It may only be a minor problem now, but it keeps you awake. Not sleeping can create new problems.

"I've tried everything..."

When you come to a dead end after trying everything, and nothing seems to work, it could be time to investigate an alternative. Many of my clients have been there and are now sleeping peacefully.

Many doctors today will recommend lifestyle changes as part of a more holistic treatment for chronic disease or common diagnoses. Pills are easy to take but improving habits that helped us to get sick in the first place can be harder to change. Together we look at these questions:

Why is it so hard to implement strategies I know will help ease my sleeping problem?
Have I just given up because it's all too hard?
Is it a case of letting life take priority over my needs?

Your health is worth saving. Brain Coaching will help renew your feelings of self-worth, develop positive neural pathways that will support you in taking care of yourself, and motivate you to implement good health and sleep hygiene strategies. You are not alone.

CHAPTER 7

Psychological/Emotional Issues that Influence Sleep

"Neuroimaging and neurochemistry research shows that good sleep helps with both mental and emotional health[1]"
Harvard Mental Health (2021)

Sleep deprivation and mental well-being are closely connected. There is a bidirectional relationship between the two - sleep loss leads to decreased mental and physical well-being, and vice versa; poor psychological and physical well-being contributes to sleep loss. Most of us can relate to how hard it is to function after a night without sleep. Many people have certainly suffered the consequences after travelling overnight, pulling an all-nighter to finish a project, staying out with friends, or being there for a sick child. We also know what it feels like to go night after night on little to no sleep - feeling 'out-of-it', trying to work in a state of confusion and apathy, hurting loved ones with snappy behaviour, beginning to hate yourself for behaving this way. Without appropriate intervention, a downward spiral of poor sleep, combined with increased emotional and physical dysfunction leads to anxiety and depression. Treating sleep loss and subsequent chronic insomnia problems is essential for creating an 'upward spiral' of good health. Treating insomnia before it leads to significant health problems, like heart issues or auto immune disorders, is more desirable. Improving sleep is also a first step towards preventing and treating psychological conditions in their early stages.

There are many reasons you wake up in the middle of the night. If you have addressed the obvious reasons, as suggested in previous chapters: environmental interruptions, inadequate diet, medical implications, and physiological factors, the remaining reasons could be emotional or psychological. Being awake in the middle of the night is nothing to be embarrassed about —many people suffer this problem.

Definition: Psychological - of, affecting, or arising in the mind; related to the mental and emotional state of a person, having a mental rather than a physical cause. (Oxford Dictionary). The word psychology derives from the Greek word psyche which means soul. The American Psychological Association (APA) defines psychology as the scientific study of mind and behaviour.

Sometimes the reason for insomnia is apparent – stress or worry about work, money, family, or relationships. Sometimes the cause is not so obvious – trauma, guilt or shame related to past or present events. Emotional reasons uncovered in my clinic, which keep people awake at night, include: guilt, shame, worry, or responsibility – whether real or imagined. Living with these feelings starts a seemingly inescapable pattern of thinking and behaviour that leads to sleepless nights. These feelings could be based on something that actually happened or could be based on something we imagined happened. We may not know the real reason for our insomnia.

Working with some of my clients, I have uncovered deep-seated habits of feeling guilty or responsible for something (or everything) of which they weren't aware. They thought they had dealt with an issue at the time, but a habit of blaming themselves and feeling bad about what happened started a habit of thinking which has never left them. Their brain developed a habit of dwelling on these feelings at 2 or 3 o'clock in the morning. Their 'monkey brain' took over, swinging from what-if to why-didn't-I, from feeling wretched to feeling hopeless. They couldn't stop dwelling on everything they needed to 'fix' in their life. We uncovered the original trigger and then resolved the issue so they could move on. Then together, we created a relaxing routine to achieve a peaceful night's sleep. The result, achieved in the Brain Coaching session, broke the habit or pattern of thinking emotionally about the past or the present and enabled logical thinking to deal with the present. Let's look a little deeper into some of the emotional factors affecting sleep:

Anxiety

Anxiety is worrying excessively about the past, present, or future. Many of us can feel anxious about being late, about what people think of us, about our performance either in the past, present, or future, or even about being in crowds. Many everyday situations can cause us to feel anxious. Feeling anxious in these situations can lead to a build-up of emotional stress that keeps us awake at night. In most situations, we can reason logically and take stock of the situation. If you have found out a loved one has a terminal illness, or your house will be repossessed, of course you will worry, but logically, there are steps to take and supports in place that can lessen anxiety. When you are sleep deprived, you are more susceptible to emotional stress, and coping with decision-making and day-to-day life becomes harder. Cherie, a young woman I worked with, anxious about work and her performance, couldn't stop fretting in the middle of the night. Her brain was in the habit of waking up at 2 or 3am and going over everything she did or didn't do the previous day and what she needed to do the next day. Her anxiety levels were getting worse each day. We resolved her issues. Logically, she knew that she couldn't do anything at 2am. We developed some mindfulness tools to help her feel calm, and she now sleeps through the night. She said she is so relieved!

Depression

Depression is extreme sadness or despair that lasts for more than a few days. We constantly feel bad or sad or lack interest in daily life. Depression feels like existing in a 'black hole' – all you feel is darkness and there seems to be no escape, no end in sight. This can feel debilitating, frustrating and is hard to break free from. Depression impacts our relationships and work. Even the most well-adjusted of us can experience degrees of depression. Logically, we would seek help when experiencing signs of prolonged depression. When sleep-deprived, we find it hard to think rationally which exacerbates the symptoms of depression. Sometimes it isn't easy to work out what comes first. Are we depressed because we are tired and fatigued? Or are we tired and fatigued because we are depressed? Either way, we can be plagued by sleepless nights. Marion was having feelings of depression (not enough for her to go to the doctor for anti-depressants – she said she didn't want to do that) and wasn't sleeping well. This started a snow-ball effect for her. She was tired and didn't get as much done in the day as she wanted to, which added to her depression and feelings of not being 'good enough'. She would then lie awake at night going over all the things she didn't do, and 'beat herself up', over and over again. This was a terrible cycle for her. After we uncovered what was causing her to feel this way, and reinforced and reminded her she was good enough, her logical thinking gradually took over. Marion used positive strategies to improve her sleep and started feeling more energised during the day, becoming even more productive. Once she felt more productive, Marion's depression lifted.

Anger or resentment

Anger or resentment produces strong feelings of annoyance, displeasure, hostility, or indignation at being treated unfairly. Feelings of anger or resentment can stem from a past incident, an ongoing conflict, or difficulties at work. These feelings can perpetuate if left unresolved, especially when we feel justified for feeling this way. If allowed to build up, the stress of feeling anger or resentment can raise cortisol levels, causing sleepless nights and further exacerbating the situation. We look for every nuance, word, or act from other parties to justify our irrational feelings. Under normal circumstances, we can use techniques like forgiveness, dismissing or ignoring other people's behaviour, or using distraction strategies, such as changing the subject or making a joke, to relieve feelings of anger or resentment. When tired or exhausted, we live on edge and the slightest upset can make us feel angry or resentful. It becomes more difficult to forgive or ignore other people's behaviour. Another client, Andrew, a hard-working young man, had trouble coming to terms with his parent's divorce. He really missed his mum and felt her loss in his life. It was as if he couldn't find pleasure in his life and was very unhappy and angry. He threw himself into his work to try to overcome his sense of loss. His emotions interfered with his sleep – he knew he had to get decent hours of sleep because he worked so hard during the day and was so grumpy with everyone around him. This only made him feel more annoyed and angrier. No-one wanted to be around him and he found fault with everyone, including himself. This young man also had psoriasis. Once we uncovered the reason for his acting the way he was, and introduced some tools to reinforce new positive habits, he started sleeping better; he felt less angry, his stress levels decreased and his psoriasis diminished. He said he couldn't believe it!

Stress

"Stress is a state of worry or mental tension caused by a difficult situation. Stress is a natural human response that prompts us to address challenges and threats in our lives. Everyone experiences stress to some degree." (World Health Organisation).

Some amount of stress is normal in everyday life. When stress impacts your life and leads to sleeplessness, it becomes a problem. Sometimes, stress is needed to get adrenalin flowing to react in certain situations. For instance, if a fire was raging towards you, a surge in adrenaline would enable you to physically move away. A certain amount of stress can even spur us on to get things done! A rational reaction to feeling highly stressed would be to implement techniques that will bring down cortisol levels and facilitate mental calm. We can leave a stressful situation, take deep breaths, ask for help, or confront and diffuse the source of the stress. If, however, we cannot turn the stress level down when there is no danger, then health issues or sleeplessness can result.

Lying awake, feeling tense and stressed and getting worked up about things that are not in our control is not helpful. We can then become stressed about not getting enough sleep! One of my clients, Fiona, had the classic symptoms of dealing with stress. She had work problems and wasn't sleeping well. Fiona was self-medicating with alcohol and consuming caffeinated drinks throughout the afternoon because she needed that 'pick-me-up.' Her family relationships were suffering, and it seemed like she was reeling from one stressful situation to another, nearly at breaking point. Fiona has now retrained her brain to cope with emotional stress when things don't go the way she wants or expects; she has given up caffeine, has cut down on alcohol and is enjoying family life. Her sleep has also improved.

Catastrophising

Catastrophising is believing that a worst-case scenario is likely to happen. We can catastrophise everyday situations – a student panicking that they will forget a speech, worrying about running out of fuel before the next petrol station, or fearing children will be hurt on the way to school. Some who tend to catastrophise will even blame themselves for something that has nothing to do with them. This is not logical thinking but, for them, it's hard to stop this line of thought. Catastrophising can even lead to panic attacks because the worry is so convincing. When we are in the grip of catastrophising, we can't think straight. Rationally, we can assess the situation and either do something about it or employ calming strategies, such as taking a deep breath or visualising a positive outcome. For others, outside intervention may be needed to assist in calming their catastrophic thinking. Heather, another client, used to often blame herself if anything happened to a member of her family, even when they lived interstate! Heather would think that somehow, she could have prevented it from happening or should have warned them. Even if nothing happened, she would worry herself sick about what could go wrong, and how she could stop it from happening. It was only after it was outlined logically that these events had nothing to do with her she could calm down, see sense, and realise that other people are responsible for themselves – they were not her responsibility.

Procrastinating

Procrastination is the act of unnecessarily postponing decisions or actions, even when we know negative consequences could result. Some of us have valid reasons for delaying decisions or activities and will get other jobs done instead. Others will procrastinate to their own detriment, even delaying their bedtime! Putting off things we know we should do can be counter-productive, not finishing a project by the deadline can result in missing out on a promotion, etc. There are psychological reasons people procrastinate. Some have such a sense of perfectionism, they will not start a task if they can't do it perfectly. If there is a history of failing at tasks, tasks will not be started to avoid defeat. Some of us use technical devices or games until all hours of the night instead of going to bed at a reasonable hour, upsetting our sleep routine. Logically, we can get the job done without procrastination. If we are sleep-deprived, tasks can seem that much harder to complete. I have had clients who procrastinate about all sorts of issues in their life: whether to go for a job interview, to sort a family breakdown, or even whether to go to bed at a reasonable hour. Some of my clients say that prior to bedtime is the only time they get for themselves - that is their 'me time' and so, they read, watch TV or play games or use social media until the early hours, even though logical thinking tells them they will be valuing themselves more if they allow themselves to get a good night's sleep. Using Brain Coaching, we work through this need to stay up late, and put in place mindful, relaxing strategies that create a reward for getting into bed by a reasonable hour.

Self-doubt

Self-doubt is the tendency to question our competence, self-worth, and performance. As self-assured people, we readily accept ourselves and our capabilities. We can judge whether we need to improve our performance rather than stressing or berating ourselves. When we slip into self-doubt, we second guess ourselves so much it can keep us awake, threatening our emotional stability. We keep going over and over all our perceived wrong-doings or failings. Sleeplessness only serves to perpetuate these feelings. When we are well-rested our emotional well-being is more stable, and we can feel content and more accepting of ourselves.

James, a middle-aged client, the kindest, most caring person you could ever hope to meet, was so full of self-doubt that it kept him awake at night. He worried he was not looking after his family as well as he should be. After working on irrational thoughts and what he can do about them, James now sleeps seven hours per night, regularly.

Over-stimulation

Over-stimulation is when our senses take in more information than our brain can process effectively. Over-stimulation can contribute to higher stress levels, especially just prior to bedtime. Rationally, we have a relaxed attitude about our bedtime routine and know not to engage in activities that will excite our system. When we are over-stimulated, we are 'primed and ready-for-action', rather than feeling calm and winding down from the day's activities. A relaxing evening routine helps us prepare for bedtime, keeping in tune with our circadian rhythm. We should know that using screens in the middle of the night will not help us get back to sleep, and that it usually causes our brains to become more stimulated, making sleep even less likely. I have a young client, Emily, who has a habit of using electronic devices in the early hours to 'while away the time' until she gets tired again. As a result, she wakes up in the morning not feeling refreshed at all. Emily now has tools to use if or when she wakes up and resists using her phone or electronic device. She said it doesn't take her long to get back to sleep now.

Trauma

Traumatic events typically involve a sense of horror, helplessness, serious injury, or the threat of serious injury or death. Past trauma is difficult to get over. When we can deal with a traumatic event, we resolve emotions experienced as a result of the event and compartmentalise what happened. We can acknowledge the event without adding to the emotional toll. We don't just 'forget about it and move on'. We are only human. Of course, there will be memories of any trauma every now and then. When we are not able to process the emotional impact of a trauma, those memories can affect our life moving forward. An unresolved trauma can cause us to relive the event, going through all the turmoil and unresolved emotions, over and over. We may experience this at a conscious or subconscious level. To feel more at peace with ourselves, and sleep better, traumatic experiences must be emotionally resolved. I had a young client, Travis who, we discovered, had been in a car accident as a child. He said, "Oh, it was only minor – no-one died." But to him as a child, it was traumatic, witnessing all the emergency vehicles and not knowing what was going on, or even if his parent was going to live. Symptoms he experienced as he grew up included trouble sleeping soundly, and not being able to concentrate at school. Travis' friendships suffered as well. During Brain Coaching sessions, we resolved how he felt about the original car accident, then developed strategies focusing on how he wanted to live his life from now and into the future.

World Events

Thinking about world events - disasters, epidemics, dangerous politicians and other events outside our control, can trigger feelings of fear, anxiety, anger, or trauma, even though we may know this is counterproductive. Thinking about or worrying about a world event can set off stress reactions raising cortisol levels, causing us to toss and turn all night. Logically, there may be something positive we can do – start a campaign, write letters, or volunteer to the cause. We can decide on activities that we can influence or feel comfortable doing, rather than losing sleep over events we cannot control. We can also implement calming techniques to feel relaxed while we come to terms with what is feasible and what isn't.

> *"Circles of control – what can you control? If it is not within your control – put it aside."*

Though once we are awake, and lying there with nothing but the vast space that is our mind - every past event, present worry or future catastrophe under the sun jumps in (real or imagined; past, present, or future; big or small) to fill that space. That 'busy' brain, sometimes called 'monkey brain'*, goes into overdrive and conspires to keep us awake. Monkey brain jumps us from one irrational thought to another – like swinging from tree to tree. This can become frustrating and exhausting. Before you know it, this perfectly natural brain function of remembering, planning, and solving problems becomes an unintentional habit of overthinking, which is hard to break. You may have tried all sorts of remedies such as adjusting your environment, improving your diet and taking medication when, what you really need, is help to get your logical brain to overcome your emotional brain.

Monkey brain is a Buddhist term meaning "unsettled; restless; capricious; whimsical; fanciful; inconstant; confused; indecisive; uncontrollable", it is suggested that it is your inner critic, not letting you rest or to be at peace. Calm the monkey brain by using mindfulness techniques, deep breathing, and/or binaural beats music.

It is not logical to lie awake for hours ruminating over the past or worrying about the future, about things you can't ever change. So why do we do it? We know it's not good for us – mentally or physically. But it can become a habit that is hard to break.

Brain Coaching helps to change your debilitating emotional habits, replacing them with positive, logical, sleep-restoring habits. Like anything new, it takes time to reinforce new habits and develop new neural pathways. Once new habits take hold, you will sleep through the night or at least get back to sleep easily if you do wake up.

Continued bouts of sleeplessness can lead to anxiety and depression[2]. And anxiety and depression can lead to sleeplessness. It is important to address your sleep issues or seek professional help if you experience symptoms of depression. About 75% of people who have depression also have insomnia. And about 40% of people who have insomnia also have depression. Not all people with sleep problems will have depression, (www.SleepFoundation. org). Again, please consult your medical practitioner for a more accurate diagnosis.

Role of REM and non-REM sleep in helping to reduce anxiety:
Sufficient, quality REM sleep is important for reducing anxiety and regulating emotions so that we don't experience extreme emotional highs and lows. There have been many trials over the years studying this connection. The relationship between REM sleep and anxiety works in reverse – reduced anxiety leads to good quality REM sleep[3] while less REM sleep can lead to increased anxiety. During REM sleep, the brain stores memories and resolves anxieties, while non-REM (slow wave) sleep helps the body regenerate cells and fights off infections, promoting positive health. Both non-REM and REM sleep have a role to play in restorative sleep. Refer to previous chapters on REM sleep for more detail.

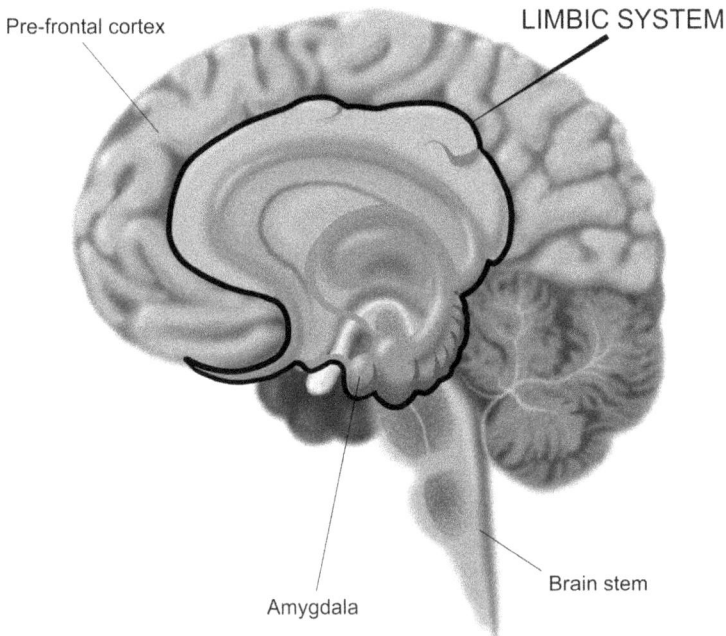

Role of the amygdala – our emotional brain
Original Artwork: Graeme Compton

Definition: The amygdala is a small, almond-shaped structure inside your brain. It's part of a larger network in your brain called the limbic system. When it comes to your survival, your amygdala and limbic system are extremely important. These are parts of your brain that automatically detect danger. They also play a role in behaviour, emotional control, and learning. (Cleveland Clinic – Neuroanatomy 2022)

The amygdala (ah-mig-da-la) is a part of the brain where emotional memories are stored. When something stressful or traumatic happens to you, e.g. if you're in a car accident, the memory of that event is stored in the amygdala. When the stress and trauma associated with the accident is logically and reasonably processed, at the time, the emotional aftermath of that event is reduced. You won't forget that it has happened, but its impact on your life will soon fade. If the stress and trauma associated with the accident is not logically and reasonably processed, the memory of this event becomes a trigger when stress is experienced later. The reaction to the trigger manifests in different ways for different people. One of my clients, Michael, was bullied at a young age. Later in life, he developed insomnia and became depressed. The trauma of the bullying started a neural pathway of thinking, reinforcing that he wasn't 'good enough'. This played out across his life, from poor behaviour at school, to poor performance at work and difficulties within the family. Michael is much more calmer and has improved relationships with family and friends in recent times.

Some clients I work with have unprocessed memories stored in their amygdala which come to the fore when they are under stress. The unprocessed memories trigger unwanted reactions, including worry or stress, that keep them awake.

Studies using functional magnetic resonance imaging (fMRI) have shown that the amygdala can go into overdrive when emotions are triggered. (An fMRI scan is a scan that measures and maps the brain's activity). Trial participants experienced increased emotional reactions when shown disturbing photographs. One of these studies, from Stockholm University, compared reactions of participants who were sleep-deprived with participants who were allowed to sleep during the trial. Both sets of participants were shown negative or disturbing images, and their emotional reactions were measured[4]. The results showed that the people who could sleep had less emotional reaction to the photos. The pre-frontal cortex of the brain is where logical reasoning takes place. It lets the brain know whether the threat (from the images) is real or not. In sleep-deprived participants, the amygdala (emotional response area) took control of the pre-frontal cortex and logical reasoning was harder to implement.

In a Tel Aviv University study[5] (2015) the results agreed with the above study – *"Insomnia makes the amygdala unable to regulate emotions and allocate brain resources necessary for objective cognitive processing."*

This is the action that is corrected and strengthened during Brain Coaching. We encourage the logical part of the brain to take over from the emotional part of the brain, subsequently reducing the emotionality of the issue, reducing stress levels and making a relaxing sleep more likely.

A lack of beneficial REM sleep contributes to a snowballing effect of negative, confused and even tortured thinking. Emotional thinking spirals out of control – we are less grateful for what we have, our relationships suffer, and our physical health declines.

Your insomnia might be relatively recent, or it could be years old. It is not too late to change this habit. The brain has plasticity (see box for definition) allowing you to correct and change your thinking habits. Can you identify the reason that you are lying awake for hours on end - the 'Why'? You can move on when you identify the 'Why' and resolve that cause.

> The Encyclopedia Britannica describes **Neuroplasticity** *"as the capacity of neurons and neural networks in the brain to change their connections and behaviour in response to new information, sensory stimulation, development, damage, or dysfunction"*.

CASE STUDY

Danielle had extreme general anxiety. Everything about her day caused her anxiety. Once Brain Coaching resolved the reasons for her anxiety, Danielle could then implement daily stress relief exercises, her sleep improved from four hours per night to seven to eight hours, and she could put herself back to sleep even if she did wake up. Then, once her sleep improved, her anxiety levels decreased. This subsequently had major flow-on benefits into other areas of their life. Danielle was very happy and relieved. Previously Danielle had such severe anxiety that she had had suicidal thoughts. *"I am so grateful for Brain Coaching. It improved my sleep, and that wasn't even the original reason that I came to Brain Coaching in the first place!"*

When the reason for insomnia is not so apparent. Brain Coaching techniques identify the real reason for sleeplessness. It might not be what you expect! Many of my clients can put themselves back to sleep when they wake during the night, instead of staying awake for hours.

They now realise that they can do nothing about the situation in the middle of the night. Brain Coaching helped them identify their issue and developed strategies that suited their situation. Another client, Sarah, told herself that she was comfortable with 'a bored mind' in the middle of the night, instead of a 'busy mind'. Once this became her new habit, she resumed sleeping seven to eight hours each night. Better sleep will help you deal better with life's stressors.

Proactive Emotional Strategies

Mindfulness: A Powerful Tool

Mindfulness is, *"a mental state achieved by concentrating on the present moment, while calmly accepting the feelings and thoughts that come to you, used as a technique to help you relax."* (Oxford Dictionary)

There have been many trials proving how mindfulness can help people with insomnia. Gross et al. (2011)[6], conducted a major review of sleeping trials that compared mindfulness treatments with other forms of sleep aids, including pharmaceuticals. Some studies showed comparable sleep improvement with mindfulness techniques and medications. However, when participants were interviewed, the majority indicated they would rather keep using mindfulness techniques than drugs, mainly because of the potential side effects of continually taking medications.

Mindfulness has gained popularity as a powerful tool to reduce anxiety and depression, lower blood pressure and improve sleep. Mindfulness calms the nervous system, switches off the 'fight/flight' reaction, and brings the body into a relaxed state. By practicing mindfulness consistently, it is possible to alter your moods and thoughts, allowing you to sleep better.

A systematic review by researchers at the National Institute of Health, USA,[7] (2019) shows that mindfulness significantly improved the quality and quantity of sleep. This resulted in improved mental and physical health. Longitudinal studies by Gross et al. [6] (2011) also found that mindfulness treatments reduced insomnia and improved other sleep outcomes in people with mental health disorders.

Sharma & Rush[8] (2014) found that mindfulness increased sleep quality and reduced stress, improving memory. It has even been suggested that it may offer some protection against Alzheimer's.

Here are some easy ways to bring mindfulness, and all its benefits, into your life:

- Deep Breathing.
- Concentrate on a colour that is calming to you.
- Muscle relaxation.
- Repeat a positive mantra.
- Concentrate thoughts on something positive.
- Promote 'decentring thoughts' (view thoughts as just thoughts, not as facts).
- Meditation.
- Write a gratitude journal.
- Sit in nature.
- Take a walk.
- Get creative.
- Cook.
- Worry times – have set 'worry' times during the day, knowing that daytime is the time to spend on these issues, not in the middle of the night.

- Instead of a 'Busy' brain, or 'monkey-brain', in the middle of the night, opt for a 'bored' or peaceful brain instead.
- Consider what exactly is in your sphere of control. Ask yourself, '*What can I control?*'.

Writing a gratitude journal before you go to sleep can also help regulate emotions. Being mindful of all the good things in your life just before going to sleep is a lot better than thinking of all the things that have gone wrong or may go wrong in your life. Buddhist monks have a mindful practice thinking of 1000 things to be grateful for, but three things per day is a good start for the rest of us!

Mindfulness shifts our brain from problem-solving (busy) mode to just 'being' mode or quiet mode. Focusing on feeling grateful for all that's positive in our life instantly calms us, reduces cortisol levels, improves our outlook, and subtly rewires our brains. Performing mindfulness activities at bedtime prepares us for sleep.

A comprehensive, longitudinal research study by Desbordes et al.[9] (2012), found through functional Magnetic Resonance Imaging (fMRI) that mindfulness had a direct effect on the brain and can affect the processing of emotions in everyday life. They found it occurred not just during meditation or the conscious act of being mindful but had a long-term effect. Interestingly, there was no difference in emotional activations or reduced anxiety in their control group, where only health was discussed, and no mindfulness practices took place. So, just talking about problems and emotions didn't make any difference to their anxiety levels. The difference was mindfulness. Even beginners practising mindfulness see benefits in a short time.

Jon Kabat-Zinn, creator of the Mindfulness-Based Stress Reduction (MBSR) program, says that mindfulness lights up parts of our brains that are not usually lit up when we are mindlessly lurching from one 'important' chore to another[10]. Kabat-Zinn defines mindfulness as: *"the awareness that arises through paying attention, on purpose, in the present moment, non-judgementally."*

You can be mindful in any situation. Being mindful is a choice. When you consciously choose to be mindful daily, you naturally retrain your brain. Practicing mindfulness daily becomes easier and easier. It is a powerful tool.

Being mindful in everyday situations means being aware, slowing down, not judging yourself (or others), paying attention. It is amazing how much you can learn and improve yourself when you become more mindful. Your relationships improve, and you are kinder on yourself. And when you engage in mindfulness activities to help your sleep problems, you'll see instant improvements. Because you are less judgemental of yourself, worrying less, even thinking more logically, you can relax and calm yourself back to sleep.

> *"Multiple meta-analyses of mindfulness-based interventions support improvements in stress, mood, anxiety, and pain. Research similarly suggests that relaxation techniques may be helpful for anxiety associated with medical procedures or conditions, insomnia, labour pain, chemotherapy-induced nausea, and joint dysfunction[11]."* (Luberto et al., 2020)

Meditation is a form of mindfulness. It focuses the mind on one thought and helps to clear the mind of other intrusive thoughts. It enhances a sense of calm rather than calamity. Richie Davidson[12] in his research on Neuroplasticity and Meditation said that it doesn't actually take that long to introduce this new habit and make it stick: *"We've shown in the laboratory that meditating for a half-hour a day for two* *weeks is enough to produce changes in the brain,"* he says. *"Meditation is a form of mental exercise. And once you begin to experience beneficial changes, it will inspire you to continue practicing for the rest of your life."*

Meditation has flow-on effects for both your physical and mental well-being. It has been known to reduce blood pressure, and to reduce cortisol (stress hormone) levels. It can also help to reduce levels of pain. Meditation can also influence emotional well-being by reducing stress and feelings of anxiety. It also helps you become more accepting of yourself and those around you. It helps you to be kinder and more empathetic. Meditation has powerful, effective, and rewarding results when combined with deep breathing. Think of it as a very inexpensive form of therapy.

It is recommended that beginners use guided meditation to get started. This can be an in-person guide or a guided meditation app. They will take you through the basics of meditation and explain why and how to do it for best results.

Even 7 minutes of meditation per day is beneficial, then gradually build up to 20 – 30 minutes. There are 1440 minutes in one day. 7 minutes is 0.05% of your day. Can you spare 7 minutes? You still have 99.95% of your day to do other things!

Below is a list of the most popular types of meditation. It is best to try them for yourself to see what works for you.

- Mindfulness Meditation - paying attention to just one thought, focusing on one positive thought, and/or focusing on your breathing. When you drift off to other thoughts, let them pass. Come back to your one positive thought and breathing.

- Spiritual Meditation— many religions practice forms of meditation. Prayer is considered to be a form of meditation.

- Focused Meditation - involves using one of the five senses: smell, touch, hearing, sight, and taste. You could listen to the sounds of chimes or water, look at a flame or the stars, or count breaths. There are many things you can focus on, rather than intrusive thoughts. Proponents say it helps sharpen attention.

- Mantra Meditation - is used in Buddhism by using a repetitive sound, like ohm or hmmm. Or sound can be replaced with a phrase of your choice. The mantra can be repeated internally or out loud. For some people, speaking it out loud causes a vibration in the throat that can be calming as it vibrates the vagus nerve.

- Movement Meditation – some people consider yoga to be a type of movement meditation. Other types are walking, tai chi, or repetitive activities like swimming, cycling, or rowing with slow, rhythmic repetition using both the left and right side of the body – bilateral stimulation. Combine this with your positive mantra and you have a winning combination! Movement meditation involves just concentrating on your action, rather than your worries or performance.

- Transcendental Meditation - is a trademarked type of meditation taught by specialist yogi teachers. It involves meditating to a deeper level.

- Progressive Relaxation Meditation – you progressively concentrate on the muscles in your body (also known as the body scan meditation). Concentrate on one area or muscle starting at the feet, slowly tightening and releasing these muscles, then move onto the next part of your body. This helps to relieve tension and to calm down before going to sleep. (One client told me that when they did this, they couldn't get past their shoulders before falling asleep!)

- Loving Kindness Meditation – by repeating phrases of love and acceptance to both yourself and to others, this meditation promotes a sense of acceptance and gratitude by dispelling negative feelings. Concentrate on the good things about a person rather than their bad points (this goes for yourself as well!). This meditation will have a flow-on effect to other parts of your life. It may even relieve tension enough to allow better sleep without resentment building up.

- Visualisation Meditation – as the name suggests, you visualise or imagine a calm and peaceful setting. Use all your senses if you can, like smell or touch, in this visualised scene. It can be used not only to feel calm but to imagine being successful at achieving your goal. For example, imagine starting each day refreshed, regenerated, and ready to take on the day more positively after a good night's sleep.

Zen proverb "You should sit in meditation for 20 minutes per day – unless you are too busy, and then you should sit for one hour"!

BUT!!! – I hear you say …

"My mind keeps wandering whenever I try meditation."

Brain Coaching helps bring your mind to a calm state, then supports you to establish positive habits, like mindfulness, until you can fall asleep.

"I don't believe in that stuff."

Perhaps there are other therapies you have tried, and they didn't work. Brain Coaching works. Many of my clients are happily sleeping through the night after we learn to relax. It can't hurt to give it a go.

"I've always been like this." "I deserve to be punished for what I did in the past." "I can't let it go."

We can deal with your past and show you a way forward that will bring peace of mind.

"I might lose my job, my family, etc."

We can't control external life events, but being awake at 2am, thinking about something that may or may not happen, will not help. Getting a good sleep is going to put you in a much better frame of mind to deal with whatever life throws at you. Brain Coaching teaches you skills to deal with life events.

"This person annoys me so much. They are awful, they're a bully."

There are strategies and tools that help you deal with difficult people. It's time for you to take back control.

Are you ready for good sleep?

Are you ready to improve your life, relationships, productivity, health, skin?

It's your time to get proactive, change your mindset; and learn new ways to sleep well.

Chapter Summary

Wouldn't it be great if we, as individuals and as a society, could treat mental health disorders early on, by improving sleep patterns, without resorting to medications? (Relying on medications only masks the problem and can lead to addiction and loss of efficacy). Treating mental health disorders before they escalate would be more cost-effective by treating insomnia earlier. Of course, not all mental health disorders will be solved by a good night's sleep, but studies have shown that sleep disruptions are a fair indicator of other developing problems.

Scientists at Pittsburgh University have found that *"Sleep complaints and depression are bidirectionally related"* [13]. A Sheffield University sleep study (2021) meta-analysis also found that *"Insomniac patients were four times likely to develop depression"*[14]. If health practitioners and therapists could use sleep as a form of therapy, society would without doubt benefit.

Brain Coaching consultations include mindfulness practices suited to you and your needs. When you have exhausted all other avenues and find nothing is working for you, and you are ready to break free from the consequences of unsatisfactory sleep, it could be time to join me for a Brain Coaching session.

My clients have broken free from their downward spiral of worry, stress, insomnia, unhappy days, and worrisome nights. Brain Coaching begins your upward spiral, where the benefits keep building on each other, and life is great.

Benefits of Activities that Support Emotional/Psychological Well-being:

- Less reactivity to stress in your life.
- Calmer temperament.
- Increased focus.
- Less anxiety.
- Improved memory.
- Balanced emotions.
- Improved relationships, professional & personal.
- Inner peace – 'liking yourself'.
- Increased productivity during the day.
- Improved sleep during the night.
- More affordable than pharmaceuticals.
- Fewer side effects than other treatments.

"Isn't it funny how problems seem to go away after a good night's sleep?" Or not seem so insurmountable?

CHAPTER 8

Children, Teenagers & Older People

"Whoever said sleeping like a baby has obviously never had one!"
(Anon Facebook)

The sleep needs of people change with their age. While infants need to sleep for half a day, adults need less sleep. In this chapter, you will learn how much sleep you need, based on your age, and why it matters. Until we turn 25, the age at which our brains are fully mature, sleep is important for the healthy development of both grey and white matter. As Tarokh et al., explain in their 2016 paper: *"The grey matter is the area where the actual "processing" is done whereas the white matter provides the communication between different grey matter areas and between the grey matter and the rest of the body"*[2].

Grey Matter: *serves to process information in the brain. Structures within the grey matter process signals generated in the sensory organs or other areas of the grey matter. This tissue directs sensory (motor) stimuli to nerve cells in the central nervous system, where synapses induce a response to the stimuli. (www.news-Medicalnet.net - What is grey matter?)*

White Matter: *Long thought to be passive tissue, white matter affects learning and brain functions, modulating the distribution of action potentials, acting as a relay and coordinating communication between different brain regions.*[1]

Children

It's no secret that the brains of humans develop from day one of conception, and then from birth, the development is exponential, especially in the first two years of life. Sleep is essential for this process. It is so important for babies, children, and teenagers to get the required amount of sleep. Good quality and quantity of sleep are vital for developing brains.

The optimal amount of sleep for a child's brain function (American Academy of Pediatrics):

- 4-12 months old = 12 to 16 hours per day (including naps).
- 1-2 years old   = 11 to 14 hours per day (including naps).
- 3-5 years old   = 10 to 13 hours per day (including naps).
- 6-12 years old   = 9 to 12 hours per day.
- 13-18 years old = 8 to 10 hours per day.
- 19 years plus   = 7 to 9 hours per day.

Babies have yet to establish a circadian rhythm, so it is essential to start a routine of sleeping at night and being wakeful during daylight hours. While they are sleeping, a lot of action is going on in their brain! Not only is the brain developing, but it is also growing in size. The baby's brain doubles in size in the first year. Memories are being stored, and synaptic connections are being made. Babies are constantly learning about the world around them, and the information is processed and stored while they sleep. The information stored becomes an essential reference for the rest of their lives, especially when learning to regulate emotions or moods. Getting the sleep/eat/play routines settled as soon as you can is important. Babies, toddlers and young children need the consistency of regular sleeping patterns for optimal brain development. Whole books have been written about babies and sleep, so I won't go into detail here.

Teenagers

Studies have shown an increase in grey matter in the brains of teenagers who get more average sleep than teenage brains with less or interrupted sleep. Taki et al. (2012)[3] conducted MRI scans on teenagers having a full night's sleep and teenagers with interrupted sleep and found a positive correlation on the amount of grey matter; the more sleep they get, the more grey matter is developed. While Telzer et al., (2015),[4] found a correlation linking the rate of white matter development in sleep-deprived adolescents compared to adolescents who were not sleep-deprived. This area of research is continuing to expand.

All is not lost! If a child has many nights of insomnia, or if you, yourself, had poor sleeping habits as a child, processing and communication in the brain can be improved by improving your sleep now. It's important to be aware of what is happening in your teenager's life that is disrupting their sleep and focus on the things that will improve their wellbeing.

A teenager's body clock, or circadian rhythm, is slightly different because their body tells them to go to sleep later at night and wake up later in the morning. Teenagers need between eight to ten hours of sleep per night, compared to adults who need between seven to nine hours per night. Research shows this is about an hour's difference on average. Even though their body clock is skewed to a later bedtime and their melatonin kicks in later, they still need at least eight hours of sleep for normal brain development and regulating emotions.

Good quality sleep is essential for the maturing of teenage brains. When they're not getting enough sleep, this process is held back or delayed. Chronic sleep loss can have troubling impacts on their daily life, and problems may arise like: mood disorders, poor decision-making skills, reduced memory and difficulty learning, or relationship issues. A lack of sleep affects: mental health, school performance, risky behaviour, diet and digestion, truancy, and self-esteem. Teenage brains aren't mature enough to always make informed, logical decisions and/ or resist peer pressure, especially when sleep deprived.

Poor behaviour resulting from sleep loss can be confused with other disorders and children can be misdiagnosed. Being over-tired and grumpy, angry, non-communicative and/or demonstrating bad behaviour might be implicated in an ADHD diagnosis. Alternatively, poor sleep and subsequent behaviours can mask a true disorder, which could be attributed to lack of sleep. In either case, it is important for children and teenagers to get good quality sleep each night.

There is also a connection between the co-morbidity of sleep deprivation and mood disorders like depression, loss of impulse control, anxiety etc. That is, a number of teenage patients with these disorders also have sleep problems.

Sleep regulation can be an effective and inexpensive therapy compared to pharmaceuticals or other expensive interventions for behavioural or emotional problems in children and teenagers.

In every generation in history, being a teenager's been hard. It's already difficult enough, learning their way in the world, and discovering how they fit in. They now have to cope with modern-day problems like social media, pressure for careers, extra-curricular activities, and world events. The more sleep they get, the better they will be able to cope.

As parents, we aim to educate our teenagers on how important great sleep habits are before problems develop or bad habits become the norm. Bad habits, like using screens till 2am, can lead to waking up irritable every day, dropping out of school, relying on medications, poor dietary decisions, or risky behaviour patterns (drink driving, smoking, taking dangerous risks).

In short, the more consistent quality sleep teenagers have, the better for brain development and maturity.

Some strategies for happy, healthy, well-rested teenagers:

- Adults discuss ideas rather than argue with them.
- Give teenagers plenty of notice for upcoming events.
- Try to avoid early morning appointments.
- Check their daily/weekly commitments – are they doing too much?
- Encourage a relaxation technique prior to bed (even 10 minutes per day is better than nothing).
- Try for an extra thirty minutes of sleep per night.
- Try the normal sleep hygiene methods as listed for adults - no stimulants prior to bed, no screens.

BUT!!! - I hear you say -

"They need their phones at night!!!"

They need to sleep at night. Do you need help negotiating a better sleep routine with your child?

"They have training at 5 am!!!!"

Can you negotiate an earlier bedtime? Can you change the commitment by discussing priorities?

"They live so far from school; they have to get up earlier!"

Sometimes situational logistics can be tricky. I can help you both make the best of a tricky situation.

"My children have to fit in with my schedule."

This is a big issue! Brain Coaching can help you sort priorities and develop strategies that will help all involved.

"They have health problems that keep them awake, i.e., tonsils, adenoids."

Can your doctor suggest solutions? Brain Coaching can help establish beneficial routines.

"They have nightmares that keep them awake."

We can identify the reasons for nightmares. Let me help bring relief to your concerns and worries.

How can Brain Coaching help teenagers?

Brain Coaching can help build motivation and develop strategies to encourage teens to put away their screens at night, to be in bed at a reasonable hour, and so much more. Brain Coaching helps teenagers boost their self-esteem and focus determination to make choices that are right for them, and not give in to peer pressure. Brain Coaching helps children and teens develop good habits – both mentally and physically.

CASE STUDY

Alex, a 17yo girl, living in the city, was extremely anxious, had frequent panic attacks, vomiting, sleeplessness, was studying to excess, making poor food choices, and was not socialising.

Alex was on the verge of collapse. She also thought that no-one else had feelings like this. She didn't talk to anyone about her problems. Alex was using electronic devices till the early morning hours, then found it hard to wake up in time for school. Because she was tired, she made poor food choices, and either didn't eat or ate junk food.

Alex sometimes missed school because she was tired and got sick frequently, which added to the pressure of keeping up with study. Then she would study for hours on end, even though she was tired. Her study time was not efficient, because her understanding and comprehension were compromised. Her parents could only watch on in exasperation because she wouldn't listen to them or follow their advice, even if they were brave enough to offer it! Plus, she didn't tell them everything. This situation also led to family arguments. No-one was happy.

Then Alex became anxious about her schoolwork and what she would do if she failed, and she felt anxious about her friendship group. She also began having panic attacks at school. She was worried about her body image because she wasn't eating enough and not exercising. Everything was just building up until something had to give.

Previously, both Alex and her parents had decided against taking medication, mainly because they both had an idea that the problem was because of the amount of sleep Alex was getting.

Eventually, she agreed to try Brain Coaching. It was a revelation to her to find out that other teenagers felt like she did. She was not alone. She couldn't believe that other people felt the same.

How did Brain Coaching help? Together, we worked on her motivation to get more sleep and follow through with various strategies that would encourage more sleep. We identified the original trigger for her behaviour. It was a combination of bullying in year seven by bigger kids, and a domineering parent. We resolved the bullying issue and devised strategies to improve her relationship with her parent. We also developed strategies to deal with the pressure of schoolwork and improve her nutrition which made her feel comfortable.

At last, she had found relief, and she had a plan that she could work on. Little by little, Alex started sleeping longer and began to feel good about herself, building her confidence. She was doing it for herself, not for someone else.

Note: I have seen many teenage clients with similar concerns to the above story. They all feel they are the only ones going through turmoil and don't know how to discuss it. They seem surprised to find out that other people can feel like they do.

Below are some interesting statistics from the Australian Institute of Health & Welfare Sleep Survey, (Nov 2021). Note the percentages for insomnia for the 18-24 age group. Also note the percentages of sleep problems for people in the 45-64-year brackets.

Table 1: Average sleep duration and prevalence of sleep problems by age [10]

Age	Sleep time hrs	Short sleep%	Poor quality sleep %	OSA %	Insomnia %	Restless legs %
18-24	7.2	13	22	5.0	26	20
25-34	7.1	14	24	4.9	18	16
35-44	7.1	20	26	3.6	16	15
45-54	6.8	22	29	12	21	22
55-64	6.9	24	25	13	23	17
65-74 +	7.0	9.2	20	12	18	17

OSA = obstructive sleep apnoea. Note: sleep time refers to average sleep duration for working nights. Source: Adams et al. 2017b; Wilkins 2016.

Older People

As our population ages and more people are over the age of 65 than ever before, we can expect an increase in age-related health issues. Health problems as we age can contribute to sleep deprivation, and vice versa - sleep deprivation can lead to health problems. Poor sleep can reduce an older person's quality of life and increase the need for personal care.

Sleep problems in the elderly population are usually more common than in younger adults. This could be due to a variety of worries or fears. Older people worry about their future and deal with loneliness, health, and mobility. They may have an increasing number of health issues to deal with, like: bladder issues, arthritis, sleep apnoea, fear of falling over, and fear of a heart attack. Their physical fitness is no longer as great as it once was. They may fear for their safety, and no one being around to hear them. They may be dealing with the side-effects of medications. These fears can keep them awake.

Addressing any possible underlying medical or environmental conditions is necessary when considering how to resolve insomnia in older people. It's also important to check whether insomnia could be masking any health issues.

The fact that a person is getting older doesn't mean that they will develop insomnia. Many older people sleep well. However, it is a natural part of human biology that we will gradually deteriorate as we age.

As we age, the sleep phase in the circadian rhythm moves forward. Hormones are released earlier at night, making older people sleepy earlier in the evening and making them wake earlier. This change in their cycle is the reason some older people have daytime naps, because they have woken earlier in the morning.

Common medical problems that can cause sleep disruptions in older people, as listed by Geriatrician Dr Leslie Kernisan[5,] are:

- Heart and/or lung problems.
- Reflux, heartburn.
- Arthritis, and other painful conditions.
- Bladder issues.
- Depression or anxiety.
- Neurodegenerative disorders, e.g., Parkinson's, Alzheimer's.

- Medication side-effects.
- Sleep apnoea, snoring.
- Restless leg syndrome.
- Sedative misuse.

Treating any of the above conditions could lead to an improvement in sleep. Poor sleep can exacerbate the degeneration of brain cells, leading to memory loss and confusion, possibly due to the disorders mentioned above, which can contribute to further anxiety. Anxiety in older people is quite common. Intervention can help put them back on the right track and lead to a more fulfilling life.

It is important for older people to keep active in mind, body and spirit by spending time out in the sunshine; keeping up good nutrition; exercising to their ability; maintaining a healthy social life; and putting security first so they feel safe at night, or when on their own. Following good sleep hygiene still applies to older people. Older people, or those close to them, can implement a range of strategies to help allay fears, ensure physical safety, and promote enjoyable and stimulating activity.

Strategies could include:

- Timetabling exposure to sunlight daily rather than staying inside, helps oil the wheels of the circadian rhythm.
- Reducing possible trip hazards and providing handrails.
- Having a phone and a light handy at night-time.
- Investigating the interactions of their different medications. Sometimes an overlap of medications can cause sleep disruptions, as can misuse or over-use of over-the-counter sleeping aids.
- Planning regular social interaction, keeping their minds active and helping them feel part of society.

CASE STUDY

Doug was in his nineties and was feeling depressed. His anxiety was keeping him awake at night. He had high blood pressure. He didn't feel like doing anything, just wanted to sit in his lounge room all day. He had limited mobility. He was also nervous about being by himself at night. He had lost interest in all the things he used to enjoy doing. And with Covid restrictions, he couldn't visit his friends at the community centre. He had got into a vicious cycle – being anxious, not sleeping, getting depressed and losing interest in everything.

Then he heard about Brain Coaching and thought he would give it a go. *"What do I have to lose?"* Doug said.

First, we identified why he felt anxious. Rather than go into his personal reasons here, we can just say it wasn't as obvious as being robbed or getting sick. We then resolved the issue that was causing him anxiety and he started feeling better about himself again.

The next step was for him to decide what he wanted to do in his life. Considering his limitations, he came up with some ideas that he was happy to implement. For example, he enjoyed being out in the garden, going for walks, even with his limited mobility, and talking to people; he enjoyed working on puzzles and listening to audible books. Soon, he started sleeping through the night. His anxiety decreased, and so did his blood pressure. His doctor couldn't believe it and asked him what he was doing! The doctor reduced his medications.

Doug is now enjoying his life.

You are never too old to change your habits. You do not have to put up with being worried or afraid. You can gain control over your situation.

BUT!!! - I hear my elderly clients say …

"I am in a nursing home."

Noise may be a factor contributing to poor sleep and even insomnia. Could earplugs be a solution? Take advantage of your close community by getting involved with activities, engaging with people you connect with, ask to be moved to the sunshine, if you aren't able to walk.

"I live by myself."

Can you spend time outside? Call your friends, join a group that can arrange transportation, enjoy activities within your ability range, organise friends, family or a community group to help improve your safety in the home.

"I have to do as I am told."

Have you asked for a second opinion? Are there friends or other experts you can talk to?

"The medications confuse me."

Can you ask your doctor or pharmacist for help? There are some clever ways to organise dispensing. If confusion is a possible side-effect, consult your doctor immediately.

"I can't walk."

But that won't keep you down! Create your own upper body exercise routines, wheel around the neighbourhood, or the garden.

Brain Coaching can help reduce the impact of emotional fears and worries, increase your confidence and motivation, and help you identify what you really want to do in your life, regardless of your age.

Alzheimer's disease (AD)

Alzheimer's is one type of dementia of the brain that causes problems with memory, thinking and behaviour. It is not a normal part of aging[6]. (American Alzheimer's Association). About 10% of the population over sixty-five will develop a form of dementia.

> Washington Uni, 2019 - *"The brains of individuals with Alzheimer's have an abundance of plaques and tangles. Plaques are deposits of a protein fragment called beta-amyloid that builds up in the spaces between nerve cells. Tangles are twisted fibres of another protein called tau that build up inside cells. Though autopsy studies show that most people develop some plaques and tangles as they age, those with Alzheimer's tend to develop far more and in a predictable pattern, beginning in the areas important for memory before spreading to other regions."*[7]

Even though genetics, brain injury, or an unhealthy lifestyle can influence the onset of Alzheimer's, recent research[7] (Washington University School of Medicine 2019) suggests that the build-up of plaque and tangles around brain cells is implicated in causing this disease. Autopsies of Alzheimer's sufferers have shown a much higher percentage of these build-ups than those without Alzheimer's. Research shows that during good quality sleep, the brain gets rid of toxic waste containing materials responsible for plaques. When sleep is disrupted or there is not enough sleep, the toxic waste is not satisfactorily excreted, and the plaque and proteins may build up around brain cells, slowly causing the eventual associated symptoms of Alzheimer's disease.

There seems to be a bidirectional relationship between AD and sleep disorders, especially as people age. People with sleep disorders have a higher chance of developing AD, and people with AD have a history of sleep disorders.[8]

Addressing sleep problems in the early stages of AD could aid the management of this disease, perhaps slowing down the progression. Sleep therapy would help the AD sufferers and reduce their reliance on carers and society. Sleep therapy can reduce symptoms of sleep apnoea and restless leg syndrome, which can disrupt sleep in AD patients.

Good sleep patterns will not reverse AD but may help reduce further deterioration in the brain.

Brendan Lucey from the World Health Organisation, in 2020, said that from 46.8 million people who had AD in 2015, this number will grow to 131.5 million by 2050, leading to an increase in suffering and a significant drain on the public health system[9]—another reason to maintain good sleep patterns.

Medication for this problem can have concerning side effects such as confusion, sedation, clumsiness, or risk of falls. Depending on a patient's situation, sleep therapy is an economical and less intrusive form of treatment.

Chapter Summary

Good sleep is important at any age, from 0 to 100+. It's never too late to change your sleeping habits and reap the benefits. Good sleeping habits starting at birth, help assist the development of the brain, which continues through life – regenerating cells, improving memory and regulating emotions. These are all important activities at any age, whether taming toddler tantrums, learning new skills, coping at school, navigating teenage life, earning a living, or dealing with retirement and physical health issues as we age. We can all do better at life if we have decent sleep. Having insomnia does not mean that a person will get Alzheimer's disease (like smoking and lung cancer – not everyone who smokes will get lung cancer), but it increases your chances of onset. Continued poor sleep, or insomnia, increases your chance of contracting other health issues. All is not lost; you can rewire your brain at any age. It is possible to change your habits, to keep those neurons firing, and improve your quality of life. Implementing new sleeping habits is much cheaper and more convenient than addressing the problems that may arise because of the snowballing effect of getting by on little sleep.

You, your children or your elderly parents will enjoy so much more energy and life once you start seeing the benefits of improved sleep. Start making small changes now, take responsibility for whatever your situation, learn and practice some new self-regulation skills. Good sleep helps build self-esteem too, no matter how old you are. Imagine your child, teenager, or elderly parent going about their day with more confidence and resilience. Help is at hand if you need guidance about what to do next.

CHAPTER 9

Shift Work and Sleep

"Sleep might be the most important aspect of building a great business, and having a high-performing body." Lewis Howes

Some clients have told me that sleep loss, and other symptoms related to shift work, is like having constant jet lag. Some people get used to shift work, and others develop chronic health problems. Reduced sleep and disruptions to the body clock can also lead to dangerous Occupational Health & Safety (OH&S) issues[1].

Many studies have been conducted on shift workers and the effect years of shift work have on their health, productivity, and safety. The research has found that chronic sleep deprivation leads to obesity, depression, diabetes, heart disease, and gastrointestinal disease. The latest research indicates Alzheimer's has a higher risk of developing[2].

Note that not all shift workers suffer from the consequences of working odd hours. Younger people can adjust better than older workers[3]. The potential for insomnia increases as people age, even when not working shifts, so older people doing night shifts may experience more circadian rhythm disruption than younger people on shift work.

Shift Work Sleep Disorder

The International Classification of Sleep Disorders (ICSD10), has defined Shift Work Sleep Disorder (SWSD) as *"Insomnia during the major sleep period and/or excessive sleepiness (including unintentional sleep) during the major wake period is associated with a shift work schedule".*

Only around ten percent of shift workers get this disorder. It is important to note that SWSD can sometimes be confused with general fatigue, which is usually rectified with a few days off, and enough sleep to help the person get back on track.

SWSD is more serious than general fatigue and if you think you are developing this disorder, seek professional help. Symptoms of SWSD include excessive drowsiness during the desired waking period; insomnia when you should sleep resulting in distress or impairment in social, occupational or other waking activities; and for symptoms to continue for more than one month. Other sleep disorders and illnesses also need to be ruled out.

The National Institute for Occupational Safety and Health (USA) and Safe Work Australia,[4] recommend the following to help limit the effects of shift work schedules:

- Avoid permanent (fixed or non-rotating) night shifts.
- Keep consecutive night shifts to a minimum.
- Avoid quick shift changes.
- Plan some free weekends.
- Avoid several days of work followed by four- to-seven day "mini-vacations."
- Keep long work shifts and overtime to a minimum.
- Consider different lengths for shifts.
- Examine start-end times.
- Keep the schedule regular and predictable.
- Examine rest breaks.

CASE STUDY

Paula lives in a major capital city and is a shift worker in a high-pressure job who gets by on two hours of sleep per day, whether working or on her days off. She has become highly anxious and can't see a way out of her predicament. It's almost as if she has resigned herself to getting by on a small amount of sleep. Paula wants to help her family during her time off work, but her health and relationships are suffering because of her lack of sleep and her increasing anxiety - she gets irritable both at home and on the job. Instead of getting as much sleep as possible in her time away from work, she only sleeps two to three hours per day. While it is understandable that she doesn't want to miss any family events, the downside is that she has become highly anxious, makes poor food choices, and always feels 'hyped up'. Paula even had a panic attack at work; she is grumpy with her family and accuses them of not understanding or appreciating her. During Brain Coaching, we got to the bottom of her behaviour. When the logical side of her knows what she should be doing – why wasn't she doing it? She had worked herself into this habit of only sleeping for two hours and couldn't see a way out. Sometimes all it takes is someone outside the situation to help find solutions.

In this case, Paula decided on strategies she thought would work with her lifestyle and family. In the short term, she decided she would allow time to prepare her own lunches rather than buy junk food. She would repeat a mantra that would calm her down in stressful situations. And for the long-term, she decided she could afford to retire from that stressful job, and be able to spend more time with her family (and get more sleep).

Shift Work Sleep Disorder (SWSD) can have dangerous consequences for long-term health symptoms and personal quality of life, and on-the-job safety. Many accidents have occurred in places of employment and on the commute to and from work because of tiredness and workers not being as alert as they should be[5].

When being assessed for SWSD, workers need at least seven days of monitoring to establish sleep patterns both on workdays and non-workdays. They keep a sleep diary, and record how tired they feel at work, and on the commute to and from work. Sleep latency is also recorded - this refers to how long it takes to fall asleep, either when they go to bed or have time for a nap. The average person takes about eleven minutes, whereas people with SWSD only take two to three minutes.

Workers need to be aware of how they treat their sleep health. Workplace personnel or management need to be mindful of the effect of work schedules on people's biorhythms and ability to get satisfactory rest.

Shift workers are prone to unhealthy lifestyle choices when tired. Culpepper[8] (2010) found that shift workers *"feel the need to smoke, drink caffeine or energy drinks or alcohol to perk themselves up"*. Anecdotal stories include workers taking pharmaceuticals or other drugs to keep themselves alert, which can sometimes lead to substance abuse and addiction. They are more likely to eat junk food over healthy choices because it is more convenient and gives them an energy boost. Sleeping pills or sedatives may be helpful to increase the amount of sleep after a shift or on days off, but shift workers may still feel drowsy once they've woken up[9]. Some sleeping pills can also have side effects and lead to other long-term problems, for example, headaches, nausea, dizziness, or anxiety[10].

In our modern-day '24-hour lifestyle', where many people are contactable at all hours for work issues, some people are 'switched on' constantly, and taking a break from work is difficult. This was more evident during the Covid lockdowns, when many people worked from home, and the delineation between home life and work life was less defined. People were finding it harder to say 'no' to checking their emails, answering calls and writing reports way past an eight-hour time block.

Interestingly, on long-haul flights, pilots and cabin crew are allocated places to sleep, but in other workplaces, where long shift work occurs, having a nap is seen as 'slacking.' Having a nap at work can actually recharge your batteries and help improve productivity. Whether this nap is taken during the allocated break, or built into the shift work hours, is up to the organisation. Strategic power naps at work can be an important strategy to reduce fatigue, and encourage alertness, especially during twelve-hour shifts, which have become more common in recent years. For example: two twenty-minute naps during a twelve-hour shift, followed by bright light, and a caffeine drink, can reduce sleepiness during the next stage of a shift[6].

Also interesting, when considering circadian rhythms or body clocks, an average day shift worker will come home from work and go to bed five or six hours later. In contrast, a night shift worker goes to bed within two hours of finishing their shift, because they are tired. They are not allowing their biorhythm to get into a rise of melatonin, which encourages sleep and reduces cortisol. The night shift worker has less deep sleep and poorer quality REM sleep, which can lead to other problems like insomnia and depression. Cheng and Cheng[7] (2017) found that *"Shift workers have a higher prevalence of insomnia and mental disorders compared to non-shift workers."*

Such is the basic need for nighttime sleep, that some shift workers fall asleep on the job, either safely (in a break room) or unsafely (at the wheel). Shift workers have trouble sleeping during daylight hours, not only because their circadian rhythm and natural melatonin levels are out of step, but also possibly because of home life expectations, daytime noise and family activities.

Insomnia and poor sleep patterns should be addressed as soon as possible before detrimental habits become established and are difficult to manage and recover from.

Shift workers need to make adaptations to their lifestyle to look after their health. They need to feel motivated to stick to changes that will help them cope better with disrupted sleep patterns. Examples of lifestyle changes could include:

- Preparing healthy food ahead of time instead of resorting to convenient junk food and high-sugar food.
- Negotiating with family and neighbours for some quiet time.
- Ensuring they have enough sleep on their days off, rather than, for example, 'getting by on two hours sleep' to fit in with family or social commitments.

How to overcome negative repercussions of shift work and prevent poor sleeping habits from becoming chronic insomnia:

- Encourage good family support.
- Rewards and support at the workplace.
- Stress management training.
- Good sleep hygiene (i.e. good sleep preparation).
- Control blood pressure.
- Take naps when possible.
- Worker-friendly time schedules.
- Physical exercise during free time.
- Nutritional food choices.
- Use black-out blinds or curtains.

BUT!!! - I hear shift workers say …

"I can't change my shifts."

Is it possible to negotiate your hours? If not, you *are* able to take control of your after-work routines. Let's work together!

"I need the money."

Sometimes, the only way is the hard way, but you can maintain a modified healthy lifestyle despite your sacrifices. I can help you!

"My family won't be quiet when I am off work."

Negotiation is key. Can you come up with ideas that keep everyone happy? We can work out some strategies.

"I need to do all these other things when I am off work, so I can only sleep for about two hours."

Time management can be tricky when you come off shift work. I can help you see through the emotional stress shift work can create, and you manage your time in a way that suits you.

"I need to self-medicate or I can't function."

Have you turned to medications as a last resort to survive at your job? If you are ready for a natural alternative, let's work together to find what suits you.

Brain Coaching can help you learn to negotiate calmly and effectively when dealing with employers and family members. Brain Coaching helps you uncover strategies that will create a beneficial lifestyle for you while you work shifts.

Chapter Summary

Workers, their families and workplace management should be mindful of the impact of long shifts on the worker's health and ability to make decisions, let alone falling asleep on the job! Consider possible repercussions of doctors working 16 hours or more straight through. If long shifts, short sleep hours and insomnia continue, problems will arise, and this is more so for older workers. The impact is not just on the individual worker's health but also their relationships, safety at work, and the commute to and from work.

Many organisations are becoming aware of tiredness at work and the cost to productivity, safety, time off, decision-making, and emotional well-being. They are implementing strategies to help alleviate some of these problems. For example, some mining companies supply a bus to take workers to and from the site so that they are not driving home tired after a 12-hour shift. Other workplaces provide sleep pods on site for their staff, so they can have a refreshing nap during their break.

The more awareness of this issue grows in wider society, and the more workplace safety is improved, the better we will all be. We will have a win-win-win-win situation. The worker wins by keeping their job in a safe manner, the workplace wins by having greater productivity, the families win by having their worker come home safely and in better moods; and society wins by having less drain on the health system, and increased safety in the community.

If you know of someone – either a shift worker or an organisation that employs shift workers, consider sleep workshops on how to get the best out of yourself and your employees, and improve your sleep and productivity.

CHAPTER 10

Good Sleep Habits

"A good laugh and a long sleep are the two best cures for anything,"
Irish proverb.

A good bedtime routine is important because:

- It puts you in a calm frame of mind.
- You can be confident that you will sleep well.
- You wake up feeling refreshed.

A good bedtime routine is necessary for all ages – babies, children, teens, and adults. A good bedtime routine builds good sleeping habits.

Good sleeping habits have a flow-on effect in all areas of your life. Being more productive in your work could lead to more clients, or a pay rise. When you are refreshed and vibrant, other people enjoy your company and want to be with you. It's likely you are reading this because you are not sleeping well. Are you ticking any of these boxes?

- ☐ Are you tired of poor sleep sabotaging your life?
- ☐ Are you ready to adopt new habits that will bring you sound sleep?
- ☐ Have you given up on a good night's sleep because it's just too hard?
- ☐ Have you come to the realisation that you are worth the change?

As your Brain Coach, I understand that poor sleep leaves us at the end of our emotional rope. I know *you* know that sleep is important. I know you know you deserve a great night's sleep. I can help you wade through the excuses, the difficult home or work situations, the habits so entrenched they feel impossible to break. But before we work together, there are many tips you can try on your own.

Strategies and/or Routines

You have probably tried a few of the following suggestions along your sleep journey. If you haven't, then these are a great place to start. Choosing any of the following tips is the first step to getting your brain into the swing of a good night's sleep.

Make your room your cave! Remove distractions, including TV, phones, gadgets, and glowing alarm clocks. If you rely on an alarm, conceal it in a bedside drawer or face it away from you. Leave phones, laptops, or other electronic devices in another room. Adjust the temperature, dim the lights, pull the curtains, and get comfortable. When you are ready – lights out!

Nighttime is sleeping time. Prioritise exercise, sunlight, work, big meals, or excitable activities for daytime or early evening. Aim to eat a light, healthy meal at least 2 hours before bedtime. Go for a gentle walk if you need to move, and dim inside lights. Let your body know that things are slowing down.

Prepare Your Mindset. Relax into a calming routine by doing any or all of the following recommendations:

To-do list. Write a list of the to-dos for the next day or the following week. This will reassure your mind so if you do wake up in the middle of the night, you don't need to worry about trying to remember everything – you know you have written it down. Besides the logical you realises there is not much you can do about it at 2am! If you think of something new and are concerned that you will forget it by morning, have a piece of paper and pen by the bed, write it down and forget about it. *(Do not use your phone in the middle of the night).*

Mindfulness. Concentrate on one positive thing that makes you smile, for at least ten minutes - a much better habit than thinking negative thoughts, reliving negative moments, or catastrophising just before you go to sleep.

Repeat a positive mantra. Find or create a mantra that is meaningful to you (this is also a form of mindfulness). For example – "I am calm," or "I am relaxed," or "I am a good person". Avoid negative words, or the word 'sleep' (it will just remind you of the problem). The repetition of a positive mantra reinforces a new pathway of thinking in your brain.

Sleep Restriction Therapy. Restrict the number of hours spent in bed not sleeping! Bed is only for sex and sleep. Go to bed when you are tired. If you are tossing and turning, get up and do something completely boring, nothing that will stimulate the brain. Go back to bed. Or alternatively, some therapists suggest you should restrict your hours in bed to the number of hours of sleep that you average per night. If you are only getting five hours sleep per night, and you need to be up by 6am, then go to bed by 1.00 am. Then, each night, spend longer in bed, until you are sleeping more than five hours per night.

Warm bath. Indulge in a warm bath or shower prior to bed. Not only is this very relaxing, but it also helps to drop your core body temperature, a signal that you are ready for sleep.

Meditation music. Relaxing music helps some people. Binaural Beats music has been effectively relaxing for many of my clients. The beats are heard through alternate ears[1]. This allows the brain to cross over the left (logical) and right (emotional) hemispheres, which assists the subconscious mind in working through any problems or emotional upsets. My clients have gained enormous relief by using Binaural Beats music apps and simultaneously repeating their mantra. (Refer to my article on this topic for more insight, see Appendix E)

Deep breathing. Shallow breathing happens when we are distracted or stressed and is not conducive to relaxation. Deep breathing naturally slows and calms the whole body. Especially useful is the four - five - six method. When you can't get to sleep, breathe into the count of four, hold your breath to the count of five, then slowly breathe out to the count of six. Keep repeating until you feel relaxed. This has been extremely helpful to many of my clients.

Colour scheme. Choose a colour that is relaxing for you. Have it close by the bed, or in your mind's eye (imagination). Concentrate on this colour while you focus on deep breathing and repeat your mantra. The effect of doing these three things at once is actually occupying your brain, your cognitive resources, so there is no room to think about all the thousands of things you usually think about when you can't sleep.

Body scan. Progressive muscle relaxation technique. Concentrate on each muscle in your body, start from your toes and move slowly up your body. Squeeze or clench each muscle as you come to it, then release and relax. This helps lull your body into restfulness. Again, this act will occupy your cognitive resources and help you feel relaxed.

Sleep Apps. There are many sleep apps on the market; some are free, and others require a subscription. Sleep apps can be very calming. You can choose apps with a guiding voice, relaxing music, or the sounds of rain or waves. Find one that suits you. I highly recommend the apps featuring Binaural Beats music.

Nighttime radio shows. Some people listen to talkback radio in the early hours, which puts them to sleep! Adjust the volume to a low setting.

White noise. White noise is a constant static sound and can be found on apps, or in your own room. You might have the sound of a fan whirring, an air conditioner humming, or an app that does this specifically. White noise can drown out annoying noises so that all you hear is constant static.

Earplugs. Safety earplugs are excellent for deadening external noises.

Scents/lotions: Used in a warm bath prior to bedtime, 100% essential oils can help in a bedtime relaxation regime. Lavender and geranium are popular scents for sleep. Some people recommend using lavender oil under their pillow, or in an infuser. Some have used other essential oils such as valerian or Rescue Remedy. Treat yourself and experiment, to see which suits you.

Relaxation techniques. Any of these can be used as part of your nightly winding-down routine – a warm bath, soothing tea, gentle yoga, massage, meditation, reading a book, breathing techniques, or a combination of these activities.

Sleep diary. A daily sleep diary can be useful for helping to identify patterns, and possible triggers, for sleeplessness. (See Appendix B for a blank Sleep Diary)

Magnesium supplement: Magnesium salts in your bath or foot soak, or a magnesium roll-on, lotion, or spray takes only around 20 minutes to take effect and has been known to help.

Gratitude Journal. Some people find that writing a list of all the good things in their life they appreciate, or positive things that happened during the day, helps them have a more restful sleep. You are going to sleep with positive thoughts, rather than negative thoughts. When you fall asleep, the last thing on your mind is most likely what your brain will process during REM sleep. Let it be positive! Thinking about all the good things in life and feeling grateful for them is also a good habit to develop with children.

I hope you are feeling inspired to set up your sleep-time routine: put away the screens, choose a relaxing activity or two, and enjoy a great night's sleep.

If this feels all too daunting and you don't know where to start – start with one, make one change and build from there. If making any change is too much and you feel you need help, I'm here for you.

CASE STUDY

Brianna was only getting about three to four hours sleep a night, and if she couldn't sleep, she would get up and clean the house. During Brain Coaching, we uncovered her sense of frustration for everything to be perfect. After we worked on that issue, she came up with a mantra and a new pattern of thinking; she realised that the house didn't have to be perfect, the fridge didn't have to be cleaned every day, and so on. She now regularly sleeps seven to eight hours per night, and is, *"more relaxed, calm, and a nicer person to be with,"* she said. Her family agrees too!

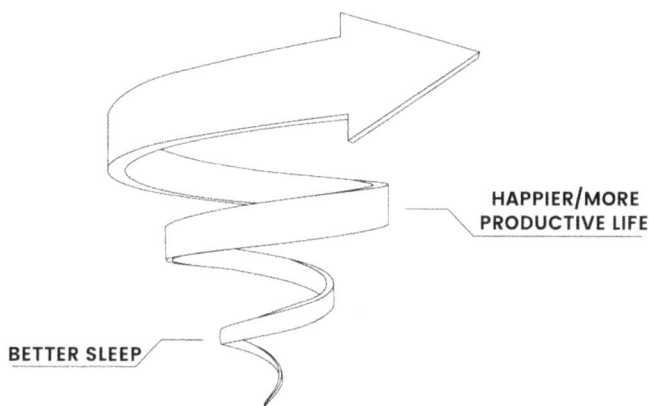

HAPPIER/MORE
PRODUCTIVE LIFE

BETTER SLEEP

GOOD HABITS

Upward Spiral

Bedtime Routine Summary:

☐ Environment – relaxing and calm, right temperature.
☐ Diet and timing of food.
☐ Supplements e.g., magnesium.
☐ Meditation/Mindfulness/Gratitude.
☐ Breathing 4-5-6 method.
☐ To-do list.
☐ Mantra.

If all else fails - GO CAMPING!! No, really! Camping covers all the bases:

- ✓ Exercise – hiking, putting up tents, collecting firewood, visiting the amenities.
- ✓ Spending time outdoors – sunshine (Vit D), fresh air, immersion in nature.
- ✓ Diet – home-cooked over the fire, no takeaway here.
- ✓ Environment – cosy sleeping bag, darkness under the sky, the quiet of night.
- ✓ Diversions averted – no screens, just the stars and a hypnotic fire.
- ✓ Gratitude.

I've heard many anecdotes and from what I have read, people say they sleep so well when they go camping compared to when they are in their own bed. I even slept all night on rocks on my Kilimanjaro trek!

BUT!!! - I hear you say …

"I feel silly repeating a mantra."

This might feel a little woo-woo to begin with, but believe me, it is not a waste of time! Persist and you will notice a difference. It is like a positive Self-fulfilling prophecy. Besides, no one but you is going to hear it.

"Writing a to-do list only makes me think of everything even more!"

Once you start to-do lists, you will never look back. You have dealt with what is on your mind and now there's room for calming thoughts. You don't need to remember things or repeat lists in your head during the night because you have written it down.

'It's expensive to get Brain Coaching."

How expensive is it to lose work because you are tired? How expensive is a break-up or a divorce? How expensive is it to have an accident because you are exhausted? How expensive is a lifetime of medications? Brain Coaching is not expensive.

Successful Suggestions

In 2022, I conducted a Sleep Survey. Below is a summary of helpful suggestions from that survey as well as what my clients and myself have tried, in order to improve sleep over the years. Some were mildly successful, and some were very successful (every individual is different). (See full survey results in Appendix C):

Sleeping tablets	Alcohol
Herbal tea	Lavender spray/ oil/pillows
Magnesium oil/tablets/bath	Acupressure mat
Melatonin supplements	Meditation
To-do list	Essential oils (various)
Therapy blanket	Mindfulness
White noise	Reading a book
Drinking warm milk	Minimise light
CPAP machine or alternative	CBD Oil (cannabis based)
Listening to boring radio programs	Muscle relaxation
Small evening meal	Repeating a mantra
Having a sleep routine each night	Journalling
Changing pillows	Ear plugs
Being so active that it exhausted them	Massage
Sex	Music, calming style
Abstaining from coffee/sugary foods/alcohol, late at night	Breathing exercises
Hypnosis	Get up until tired again
Blackout curtains	Resigning from stressful job
Brain Coaching!!!	'Not fighting' the frustration by the need to sleep

Brain Coaching could be your next step if you feel you've tried everything and you're ready to uncover what works for you.

CHAPTER 11

Brain Coaching Methodology

Brain Coaching is a process of retraining your brain, changing old negative habits into new positive habits. It is possible to retrain your brain. We identify the trigger – the elephant - and then process that trigger, so that the **'elephant can leave the room'**.

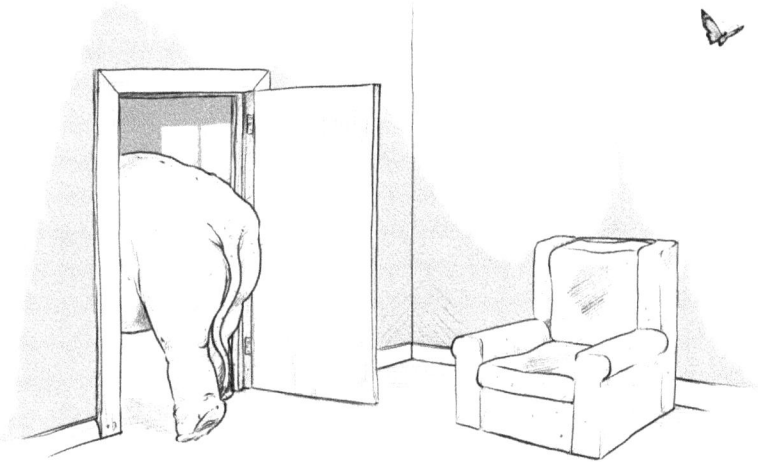

Original Artwork: Graeme Compton

The techniques used in Brain Coaching were developed by the Besser-Seigmund Foundation in Germany and have been in use predominantly in Europe and India for the past 20 years. One of the European practitioners brought this technique to Australia in 2011. Then in 2014, I completed my training in Europe.

Brain Coaching uses a combination of Myotatic Muscle Reaction Testing, Eye Movement Desensitising and Reprocessing (EMDR), Cognitive Behaviour Therapy (CBT), Neurolinguistic Programming (NLP), Mindfulness, and Bilateral Stimulation. Many therapists may use one or more of these methods, but the specific combination used in Brain Coaching makes this method so successful, generating life-changing results.

In a Brain Coaching session, I guide my client through each technique, identifying and resolving issues as we go. The client easily understands what is happening throughout the process and is then willing to initiate their new approach to life. I am there to guide them rather than tell them what they should do next, as only they know what will most likely work for them.

Identifying the Root Cause of Issues

Issues my clients bring to me include insomnia, stress, anxiety, phobias, addictions, and more. Many of my clients may have spent years putting up with disruptions to their daily life without fully realising why. They have usually sought other remedies and exhausted their search for answers before coming to see me. They may suspect it is one particular trigger causing their sleep disruption when, in fact, it is something else entirely. This isn't usually anything sinister or remarkable – but it is almost always an unresolved emotional encounter.

For example, imagine an incident that impacted a family with two children. One child coped with the experience, and the other child suffered from anxiety, resulting in insomnia. The first child could deal with and resolve their emotional reaction at the time of the event. The second child was unable to process their emotional response at the time. Instead, they continued to relive the event subconsciously. Their emotional reaction was 'stuck' in their amygdala (the part of the brain that processes emotional memories), keeping them unknowingly upset and anxious about the experience. The emotional response relating to the event was not satisfactorily processed by the brain at the time, and a combination of different factors prevented the brain from switching off, resulting in sleepless nights. Subsequent stressful events in the child's life could trigger an adverse reaction resulting in the habits of various anxious behaviours. This pattern of sleeplessness or insomnia can continue into adulthood if not addressed and resolved.

The various unresolved events or experiences, subconsciously replaying and often triggering a stress response, can vary for example: falling into a pool at a young age, humiliation or bullying, a family break-up, or a car accident. Stress can even be hereditary (epigenetic), passed down through generations. Every client's experience is different. You can escape the negative impact of past experiences.

Directed Questioning Reveals the Trigger

When my client brings their issues or symptoms, it is my job to uncover the original unresolved event or experience that triggers those unwanted issues or symptoms in their life.

It is difficult for clients to move forward without first understanding that their issue is not the issue! Sleepless nights are not the issue, they are a symptom.

In a Brain Coaching session, we begin with a focused and gentle questioning investigation. Getting to the heart of the issue relies on the client's innate response to the questions presented. The questioning continues, gently teasing out and following responses until the original event or experience is uncovered.

Resolving the Underlying Trigger

After identifying the original trigger, the next step resolves the emotional response holding the client 'stuck' in a pattern of reacting negatively to each new stress in their life.

Resolving the trigger eliminates or reduces the stored 'emotionality' of the original event or experience and allows logical, rational thinking to take its place.

For instance, imagine you lost your job. That's a traumatic event in your life – you have bills to pay, the future is uncertain, and you're facing a real-life catastrophe! Thankfully, you find another job and your life gets back on track. You have a steady income, perhaps a better income. Your bills are paid, and your family is happy. However, if the trauma surrounding your initial job loss was not satisfactorily dealt with and processed, it may continue to affect your performance in your new job. New job stressors may trigger a lack of self-confidence, a fear of failure, feelings of insecurity, panic attacks, or sleepless nights. These feelings are not rational or logical! You are back in the game with a new job – you can take care of financial and social obligations. But you find yourself acting or responding with seemingly irrational emotionality, when logically, everything is under control.

Your subconscious could still be clinging onto that feeling of being sacked and the personal blow to your self-esteem. This can lead to habitual sleepless nights. Subconsciously, even years later, you are still worrying about that feeling of whether you are good enough, but the logical you, knows that you **are** good enough. Meanwhile, that pattern of sleepless nights has developed into insomnia.

It is important to process and resolve the original trigger to be able to move on, even in times of stress, and start building new habits, including getting a good night's sleep.

In a Brain Coaching session, we use simple but highly effective methods, as mentioned earlier, that allow the brain to properly process the unresolved emotions remaining from the newly uncovered event or experience. Sitting face to face, I take my client through the gentle process of disassociating from the 'stuck' emotions, resolving them and resetting the brain. My clients feel such relief at this stage of the therapy - I can almost see a weight being lifted from their shoulders. Many have even said that this is how they feel.

Reprogramming Negative Habits for Positive Habits

After identifying the actual trigger and resolving the associated feelings, we use the brain's natural plasticity to begin developing new neural pathways – new patterns of thought to replace old patterns of thinking. Again, this is painless and simple.

In a Brain Coaching session, it's at this stage that my clients come up with their own ideas and strategies they feel comfortable implementing in their life, moving forward. I suggest many alternatives, but I do not prescribe what they should do next - they lead their own recovery strategy. They know what will suit them, and what will fit in with their lifestyle. I am there to guide and help reinforce their chosen strategies. The client will create new habits and re-train their brain on their own.

Once they start to feel more empowered and feel better about themselves, the impact of the old trigger diminishes; their stress levels decrease, they become more relaxed and better able to deal with new stressful situations. Like any new habit, perfecting this takes practice, practice, practice. Successful clients repeatedly reinforce their new habit, their new thought pattern, until it becomes their new way of thinking – their new way of being.

One of the most straightforward but most powerful techniques I use with clients to form and reinforce new neural pathways for positive thinking is the concept of a Self-fulfilling prophecy (SFP). When people constantly repeat negative thoughts to themselves, such as, *I'm never any good,* or *I'm always bad at ….., I never sleep, I'm always clumsy, I'm not good with money* – those people will never be successful because they are reinforcing the idea that they are inadequate, unsuccessful, incapable. Imagine if their self-fulfilling prophecy sounded like – *I am calm, I am a good person, I am successful at...* Saying it often and believing it results in positive changes in their lives. What they believe, they become.

If you think of an athlete perfecting their sport, they practice, visualise, and analyse their performance. A good sports person will visualise how they will achieve that perfect shot or will imagine the feeling of crossing the finish line first, until their brain internalises that way of thinking. They have created their own new neural pathway for success and being the best at their sport. This is what I help clients do to create new habits.

The Brain Coaching Method and Insomnia

Most of my clients count poor sleep or insomnia as one of the issues most disrupting their lifestyle. No matter what your sleep issue is, Brain Coaching will help. You can reclaim your sleep – it is possible.

We identify your original triggering event or experience and resolve how you've reacted emotionally to stresses. It is these reactions: worry, fear, and feeling inadequate, which keeps you awake at night. We work together to clear away these reactions.

Let me take you to stage three of the Brain Coaching session, re-training your brain. I help you formulate your own SFP (self-fulfilling prophecy), or mantra, which doesn't even mention sleep! In psychology, I learned that if you tell people not to think of a blue elephant, what will they think of? A blue elephant! If you suffer from insomnia, we will not include the word 'sleep,' because that's what your brain will think about - it will be preoccupied with whether you will have a good sleep, which is guaranteed to keep you awake!

Your ideal mantra may look like this: *I am calm, I will wake up refreshed, I will be ready for the day ahead,* or *I deserve to be relaxed.* Mantras or SFPs are customisable just for you.

We will look at ways to put your best sleep hygiene strategies in place, as mentioned in Chapter 10. Then, you design a personal sleep routine that will make you feel calmer about going to bed and ensure you sleep through the night.

You choose what works for you, and what you are comfortable implementing. My clients are amazed at how easy and effective Brain Coaching has been for them. They can make immediate changes that impact their lives in a good way! I often get a message the day following our session telling me they've slept right through – for the first time in years!

Why do Some Successes Regress?

When a previously successful client contacts me and tells me the process is no longer working, I know exactly what is wrong! Why do people fall back into their old habits? Why do they regress, especially after a period of successful sleeping? They've been going along nicely, putting their new habits into practice, then they fall back into old habits! They have stopped repeating their mantra and their other positive strategies; hence, they are not getting that internal reinforcement.

Life constantly throws challenges at us, usually when we least expect it. This may cause so much disruption and distraction in our lives that we 'fall off the horse'. We forget to keep up the practice of repeating our mantra and slip back into old habits, resulting in a return to poor sleep. When we stop or forget to keep our practice going, it's common that we receive dopamine rewards for the wrong habits! Have you slipped back into the habit of being on your screen till all hours, drinking alcohol till late, or other practices that inhibit a good night's sleep? You know these habits aren't helpful, but you can't stop doing them because you are getting that dopamine reward.[1]

Your Brain Coaching strategies will stop this unhelpful behaviour. The solution can be as simple as listening to relaxing music, taking a warm bath, repeating your positive mantra, and deep breathing, all of which feeds your 'reward' system in a good way. When you feel 'rewarded' you'll repeat this positive behaviour because it makes you feel good, and you sleep better.

CASE STUDY

One of my clients experienced regression. They were going along nicely – repeating their mantra and other healthy sleep routines that suited them, reducing their anxiety, sleeping better for the first time in years. Then they stopped all their positive habits and started sleeping only three hours a night once again. In a follow-up Brain Coaching session, we discussed why they felt that they went backward, and put them back on track again.

With any sort of training, mind or body, when you repeat a new habit and get rewarded for it, it activates all the feel-good hormones, like endorphins, serotonin, oxytocin and dopamine, and you feel encouraged to repeat it.

It's important to remember that you'll now have all the tools you need to 'climb back up on the horse' following Brain Coaching. Your brain is now wired to respond positively when using your personalised SFP or mantra. You don't always know what life will throw at you, but keeping up your positive affirming practices builds resilience, thanks to a good night's sleep.

BUT!!! – I hear you say …

"Brain Coaching? I've never heard of it!"

I'm so glad that you've read this far! Brain Coaching isn't new, but I'm one of a few Brain Coaches in Australia. If you've tried everything else, without success, is it time for you to give Brain Coaching a chance?

"How can it change my habits?"

You would be surprised how many of my clients have experienced success after sessions with me. They didn't believe it would work for them, but they gave it a chance, and their lives are now profoundly better. You'll learn just what to do for success. You are in control of your own mind.

"I've always been like this."

You don't have to put up with suffering any longer. Science has proven that the brain can develop new neural pathways, thoughts, and habits. Your life CAN change for the better.

"How can it work when nothing else has?"

This is the beauty of Brain Coaching! Many of my clients have come to me after trying every other option. Give it a try. What have you got to lose? Your sleep and your health are worth the investment.

Afterword

Why Brain Coaching?

This book shines the light on how essential sleep is to all parts of our life, at all stages of our life. Science tells us that sleep is needed to regenerate cells, improve brain function, improve emotional balance, withstand infections and diseases, and improve our ability to make good lifestyle choices. You have read about how lifestyle choices can influence sleep - bad habits to avoid, and good habits to encourage, so that a well-rested you can lead a productive, safer, and happier life.

Better sleep helps us stay safe and perform our best at work, at home, and in the community.

You are no doubt reading this book because you have problems sleeping. You may have trouble falling asleep. You may fall asleep easily but wake during the night and have difficulty getting back to sleep. You may suffer from insomnia.

Your sleep problems may have medical, physiological or environmental roots. It is recommended to consult a doctor or specialist to rule out or identify medical or physiological reasons for your disturbed sleep.

Is your sleeping environment or a lack of a sleep routine contributing to your wakefulness? When you have investigated all possible physical causes for your sleep issues, it may be time to consider whether there could be emotional reasons for your insomnia.

Brain Coaching methods help identify emotional causes for insomnia, without using medications or other expensive interventions. When it is difficult to determine the exact reason you have a sleeping problem, a Brain Coaching session can help identify and resolve a persistent past event or experience triggering a stress-based reaction. During your Brain Coaching session, you suggest strategies that will suit you and your lifestyle, because only you know what will fit in with your daily routine and other influences in your life.

Brain Coaching will help set you up for better sleep and a smoother pathway to your desired outcomes.

The next few pages have some handy reminder checklists. There is a summary of a survey I conducted with people who have or have had insomnia, revealing what has worked and not worked for them.

Try these ideas for yourself and see how you go. If you still need help to get your sleep patterns back on track, contact me at Australian Brain Coaching for an introductory chat. This is a complimentary service I offer that provides the opportunity for you to meet me in person, talk about your struggles, and explore whether Brain Coaching is the answer to your search for sleep.

It is possible to get a good night's sleep without medication. I have many satisfied clients who have come to me after having spent many years and a lot of their hard-earned money trying to improve their sleep. They have spent endless nights tossing and turning, just scraping through each day, not really enjoying life. Once they have experienced Brain Coaching and implemented recommendations, they tell me they can't believe how good they feel. They can finally get over six hours sleep and can get back to sleep if they do wake up. Some of their comments are:

"It's like a weight has been lifted."
"I am walking on air."
"I didn't know life could be this good."

Can you sense their relief and happiness? Imagine waking up feeling refreshed and ready to start the day, every day! Where will you start? A good night's sleep is at your fingertips.

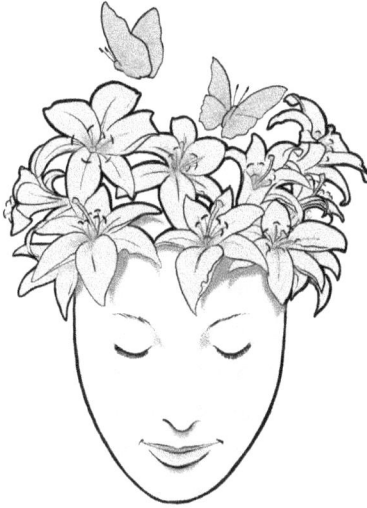

Original Artwork: Graeme Compton

Check Lists

Summary of Bad Habits that will impact on your sleep:

- Being too sedentary during the day.
- Sleeping too much during the day.
- Caffeine in the afternoon or evening.
- Having a long afternoon or early evening nap.
- Alcohol late at night.
- Heavy meal late at night.
- Screen time within an hour of going to bed.
- Too many high GI carbohydrates or too much sugar.
- Exercising late in the evening.
- Negative thoughts just prior to bedtime.
- Getting up too often during the night to go to the toilet.
- Smoking!

Summary of Good Habits that will impact on your sleep:

- Balanced diet throughout the day.
- Exercise during the day.
- Sunshine during the day.
- Quiet wind-down period one hour prior to bedtime.
- Meditation, music, and/or warm bath/shower prior to bedtime.
- Breathing exercises – 4,5,6 method.
- Repeat calming mantra.
- Practice gratitude, either in your head or write it down.
- Prepare a bedroom conducive to sleep, i.e., noise, light, temperature, comfort.
- Write a to-do list, so that it is on paper, not swirling around in your brain.
- If you wake up during the night and are still not asleep after 20/30 minutes, get out of bed and do something boring that will not stimulate your brain.
- Resist the urge to stress about going to sleep, stay as calm as you can, stop fighting it.
- Go Camping! When you are out in the wilderness, you will easily cover all the above points.

Sleep Diary

The following pages are a sleep diary. Filling it out will help you identify patterns in your behaviour and also help to keep you focused on what is essential in your life, in getting a good sleep. Because so much of your life depends on you feeling good about yourself, it is worth spending the time to fill out these sheets. This diary is fairly comprehensive as it shows just how much of our day can influence our mind and body and impact our sleep.

After a week or two, you will see what works for you and what doesn't.

You can download more of these sheets from my website www. australianbraincoaching.com.au

Sleep Diary – Mornings (How was your night?)

	Mon	Tues	Wed	Thu	Fri	Sat	Sun
Went to bed at ..pm							
Activities at bedtime *I.e, Relaxing or Stressful?							
Went to sleep at ……… - with ease -With difficulty							
Woke up at.... And again at …. And again at ….							
Got out of bed at ….							
Slept a total of …hrs							
Total time in bed … hrs							
Rose out of bed feeling – Refreshed. Somewhat tired Very tired							
Other thoughts/worries/ pain E.g., what was keeping you awake?							
During the night, any: **Helpful activities ***Unhelpful activities							

Explanation notes:

*Relaxing activities could include reading, sex, soft music, muscle relaxation, deep breathing, mindfulness, gratitude list etc. Stressful activities could include work emails, screen time, noisy setting, bright lights.

**Helpful activities during the night could include getting out of bed after 20 minutes of being awake and do something boring; or do some deep breathing, repeat a calming mantra.

***Unhelpful activities during the night could include tossing and turning for over thirty minutes; using screens; doing work tasks; using the toilet.

Sleep Diary – Evenings (Review the day)

	Mon	Tues	Wed	Thu	Fri	Sat	Sun
No. of caffeine drinks M = Morning A = Afternoon E = Evening							
No. of alcoholic drinks M A E							
No. & type of drugs M A E							
No. & Type of herbal remedies: M A E							
Amt. & Type of exercise M A E							

Daytime sleep (accidental or deliberate) mins. M A E						
#Timing & amount of last meal Carbs?						
Mood during the day						
Other thoughts/ worries/pain? i.e., prior to bed						
*Activities prior to bed: Helpful: Unhelpful:						

Meals, for example: You ate a large meal at 8pm of pasta; or you ate a small serving of roast beef and veggies with no carbs at 7pm

*Helpful activities prior to going to bed could include: Write a to-do list, warm bath, gentle exercise.

*Unhelpful Activities could include: Using screens, vigorous exercise, arguments.

Sleep Survey Results Summary

Firstly, I am very grateful to everyone who completed the sleep survey on my website. I really appreciated their time and effort in responding to the questions. Every single respondent took the time to write comments about their sleeping experiences. This information will be useful in relaying to other people what works and what doesn't (in real life), and what some of the consequences of not sleeping well look like. Their efforts and comments may help someone else to improve their sleeping habits.

The following is a brief summary of the statistics from the survey.

Q1. Regarding the question on what their sleeping problem was:

48% said that they had trouble getting to sleep,

83% said they had trouble staying asleep,

33% said that they had both problems – getting to sleep and staying asleep.

(I know this adds up to over 100%, and this is because many people said they had both problems)

Q2. The respondents said that their Average Number of hours of sleep per night were:

9% said that they got about 7 hours but that it was broken sleep and not very restful,

23% said 6 hours,

27% said 5 hours,

22% said 4 hours,

14% said that they got 3 hours or fewer, and sometimes no sleep.

Q3. Respondents mentioned certain remedies tried over the years:

54% said medication.

26% said meditation.

24% said music or some sort of calming app.

23% said other relaxation techniques.

17% said increased physical activity (even sexual activity helped).

15% said a variety of natural remedies (tea, valerian drops etc.).

(Again, these figures add up to over 100% because so many respondents used multiple methods to try to get some sleep)

Other individual solutions attempted: hot bath, counting backwards, massage oils.

Q4. Regarding the answers to the previous question, when asked "Did any of the above work?"

> 40% said nothing worked for them.
>
> 24% said that medications worked but only for a limited time.
>
> 11% said that music and meditation worked for them.
>
> 5% said that being active worked (being so exhausted that they slept), and
>
> 20% said that their own individual strategies worked, e.g., having a set routine, not having coffee or alcohol, not stressing about sleep, etc.

Q5. When asked, "Did these strategies work for long?"

> 77% said either not at all, or only for a limited time.
>
> 23% said that their particular strategy worked for years. (Note: these were mainly relaxation techniques)

Q6. Responses to the question – "How did lack of sleep affect your life?" (Many responses included multiples of the answers mentioned below):

> 56% said that they were moody/ anxious/cranky or depressed.
>
> 52% said they had lower energy levels.
>
> 41% said that they gained weight.
>
> 38% said that they were less productive.
>
> 11% said that they felt foggy in the brain.

Interestingly, only 3% mentioned that they felt more stressed. Maybe feeling anxious, moody or depressed is considered to be stressed.

Sleep Assessment Questionnaire

Australian Brain Coaching

Do you have trouble getting enough sleep?

Take this quiz to find out what are the most pressing sleep issues for you:

- ☐ Do you toss and turn during the night?
- ☐ Do you have trouble getting to sleep and/or staying asleep?
- ☐ Do you average less than 7 hours per night?
- ☐ Do you wake feeling tired?
- ☐ Do you feel tired during the day?
- ☐ Do you think that you could be more productive during the day?
- ☐ Do you make poor lifestyle choices during the day/evening? E.g., eat the wrong food? Drink or smoke too much? Don't exercise?
- ☐ Do you think that your mood could be improved? I.e., do you feel bad-tempered or grumpy?
- ☐ Do you snore?
- ☐ Do you have other health problems? I.e., autoimmune diseases; gut problems; obesity, etc.

If you answered yes to any of the above, do something about your sleep habits before it impacts on your health even further.

Brain Coaching can help put you back on the right path, without pharmaceutical or other expensive interventions or supplements.

Contact Helen to see how easy it is to start feeling better and living your best life.

Binaural Beats Music

(The following is an article I wrote in early 2020 and was reported on by a journalist for the Sunday Daily Telegraph.)

The Healing Power of Music

It's no secret that music can alter our mood, whether we listen to or play it. Loud and active is more uplifting; smooth and soft, more calming. As long ago as 1697, William Congreve wrote that music has the power to "soothe a savage breast, to soften rocks, or bend a knotted oak." Now, research has shown us we can harness these powers to create calmness and help us heal. When we are calm, we can function better, both emotionally and physiologically. This is when healing can take place.

The role of binaural beats therapy

Binaural beats therapy is an integral part of the Brain Coaching technique that I practice. It is an inexpensive, non-invasive treatment that utilises the latent power of our brains. Binaural simply means 'relating to both ears.' Binaural beats are achieved by delivering slightly different frequencies to each ear to achieve a calming tone in the middle of our brains[1]. Combining this type of music with a positive saying or mantra helps to reinforce those messages in our brain, creating new synaptic connections. It harmonises the different parts of our brains. This leads to new habits that make us more able to leave behind our old pathway of negative thoughts and behaviours.

Brain Coaching is an easy and relatively quick method of retraining your brain. It is non-threatening, non-invasive, and usually positive results can be seen in three sessions.

The stages in Brain Coaching are:

1. Identify the actual trigger for negative thoughts and behaviours.
2. Process and resolve that trigger.
3. Develop strategies that suit your lifestyle (that is, re-program your thinking habits).
4. Use binaural beats music to reinforce these new thinking habits and replace anxiety with relaxation. *(Please note- not all clients need or want this last stage, it is up to each person to decide what suits them)*.

During the Brain Coaching session, I will supply a recording of meditation music with added binaural beats (left/right beat) that you can upload to your own phone. I then help you develop your own mantra that suits your situation, and you agree to how many times a day or week you want to listen to it.

The outcome for my clients

Many of my clients have had success using this method to reduce anxiety and improve sleep. They can then come up with strategies that suit their lifestyle, personality, and situations. Clients have also noticed an improvement in concentration and performance, whether for work, creativity, exams or sports.

Sara has gone from two hours of sleep to seven per night: *"So happy. I am walking on air!"*

Marian says, *"I can recommend Helen, as I have recently been seeing her for help with insomnia. The music with binaural beats is certainly beneficial. The sessions have been very helpful and insightful."*

Christopher says, *"I loved working with you, I am more productive now. Helen is great at getting to the bottom of what is going on for you. Being able to listen to the music whenever I want is a plus. If you haven't had the opportunity to work with Helen before, now is the time".*

Esther says, *"Helen is a very experienced practitioner. I find her very approachable and her coaching has amazing results. I used her music technique to improve my concentration. I can personally recommend her whatever your concern is. Give it a go, don't be afraid, you will never look back!!"*

Emily says that she can now handle previously stressful situations and has the ability to banish negative thoughts. *"The elephant has left the room!"*

The science behind music as therapy

"Scientists have observed for decades that exposure to sound waves can affect brainwave patterns. In a process called entrainment (aka 'tuning the brain'), when exposed to sound waves at certain frequencies, brainwave patterns adjust to align with those frequencies[1]."

Scientists have been studying sound wave's effects on the brain for several years. Technology developed over the years has enabled brainwaves to be measured in response to various sounds and music. Research shows that low-frequency tones can lead to a state of relaxation. This is where music with a binaural beat can aid relaxation and reduce anxiety.

For example, scientists at the Johns Hopkins University Centre for Music & Medicine found that group singing has helped people with Parkinson's disease. They also found that music reduces anxiety and can help to reduce pain.

Binaural beat music also influences the production of different hormones, reducing the stress hormone cortisol and increasing the relaxing hormone melatonin, thus leading to greater calmness and better sleep[2].

References:

1. Alexandru, B.V., Robert, B., Viorel, L., & Vasile, B. (2009). Treating primary insomnia: A comparative study of self-help methods and progressive muscle relaxation. *Journal of Cognitive and Behavioral Psychotherapies*, *9*(1), 67–82. https://www.hopkinsmedicine.org/center-for-music-and-medicine/music-as-medicine.html

2. Padmanabhan, R., Hildreth, A. J., & Laws, D. (2005). A prospective, randomised, controlled study examining binaural beat audio and pre-operative anxiety in patients undergoing general anaesthesia for day case surgery. *Anaesthesia*, *60*(9), 874–877. https://doi.org/10.1111/j.1365-2044.2005.04287.x

List of 150 Autoimmune diseases

(courtesy Autoimmune Association, US)

A

Achalasia

Addison's disease

Adult Still's disease

Agammaglobulinemia

Alopecia areata

Amyloidosis

Ankylosing spondylitis

Anti-GBM/Anti-TBM nephritis

Antiphospholipid syndrome

Autoimmune angioedema

Autoimmune dysautonomia

Autoimmune encephalitis

Autoimmune hepatitis

Autoimmune inner ear disease
   (AIED) also known as Vertigo

Autoimmune myocarditis

Autoimmune oophoritis

Autoimmune orchitis

Autoimmune pancreatitis

Autoimmune retinopathy

Autoimmune urticaria

Axonal & neuronal neuropathy

B

Baló disease

Behcet's disease

Benign mucosal pemphigoid
   (Mucous membrane
   pemphigoid)

Bullous pemphigoid

C

Castleman disease (CD)
Celiac disease
Chagas disease
Chronic inflammatory
   demyelinating polyneuropathy
   (CIDP)
Chronic recurrent multifocal
   osteomyelitis (CRMO)
Churg-Strauss syndrome (CSS)
   or Eosinophilic granulomatosis
   (EGPA)
Cicatricial pemphigoid
Cogan's syndrome
Cold agglutinin disease
Complex regional pain syndrome
   (formerly known as reflex
   sympathetic dystrophy)
Congenital heart block
Coxsackie myocarditis
CREST syndrome
Crohn's disease

D

Dermatitis herpetiformis
Dermatomyositis
Devic's disease (neuromyelitis
   optica)
Discoid lupus
Dressler's syndrome

E

Endometriosis
Eosinophilic esophagitis (EoE)
Eosinophilic fasciitis

Erythema nodosum
Essential mixed cryoglobulinemia
Evans syndrome

F

Fibromyalgia
Fibrosing alveolitis

G

Giant cell arteritis (temporal
   arteritis)
Giant cell myocarditis
Glomerulonephritis
Goodpasture's syndrome
Granulomatosis with polyangiitis
Graves' disease
Guillain-Barre syndrome

H

Hashimoto's thyroiditis
Hemolytic anaemia
Henoch-Schonlein purpura
   (HSP)
Herpes gestationis or pemphigoid
   gestationis (PG)
Hidradenitis suppurativa (HS)
   (Acne inversa)

I

IgA nephropathy
IgG4-related sclerosing disease
Immune thrombocytopenic
   purpura (ITP)
Inclusion body myositis (IBM)
Interstitial cystitis (IC)

J

Juvenile arthritis

Juvenile diabetes (Type 1
  diabetes)

Juvenile myositis (JM)

K

Kawasaki disease

L

Lambert-Eaton syndrome

Lichen planus

Lichen sclerosis

Ligneous conjunctivitis

Linear IgA disease (LAD)

Lupus

Lyme disease chronic

M

Meniere's disease

Microscopic polyangiitis (MPA)

Mixed connective tissue disease
  (MCTD)

Mucha-Habermann disease

Multifocal motor neuropathy
  (MMN) or MMNCB

Multiple sclerosis

Myasthenia gravis

Myelin oligodendrocyte
  glycoprotein antibody disorder

Myositis

N

Narcolepsy

Neonatal lupus

Neuromyelitis optica / devic
  disease

Neutropenia

O

Ocular cicatricial pemphigoid

Optic neuritis

P

Palindromic rheumatism (PR)

PANDAS (Paediatric
  autoimmune neuropsychiatric
  disorders associated with
  streptococcus infections)

Paraneoplastic cerebellar
  degeneration (PCD)

Paroxysmal nocturnal
  hemoglobinuria (PNH)

Pars planitis (peripheral uveitis)

Parsonage-Turner syndrome

Pemphigus

Peripheral neuropathy

Perivenous encephalomyelitis

Pernicious anaemia (PA)

POEMS syndrome

Polyarteritis nodosa

Polyglandular syndromes type I,
  II, III

Polymyalgia rheumatica

Polymyositis

Postmyocardial infarction
  syndrome

Postpericardiotomy syndrome

Primary biliary cholangitis

Primary sclerosing cholangitis

Progesterone dermatitis
Progressive hemifacial atrophy
  (PHA) Parry romberg syndrome
Psoriasis
Psoriatic arthritis
Pure red cell aplasia (PRCA)
Pyoderma gangrenosum

R

Raynaud's phenomenon
Reactive arthritis
Relapsing polychondritis
Restless legs syndrome (RLS)
Retroperitoneal fibrosis
Rheumatic fever
Rheumatoid arthritis

S

Sarcoidosis
Schmidt syndrome or
  Autoimmune polyendocrine
  syndrome type II
Scleritis
Scleroderma
Sjögren's Disease
Stiff person syndrome (SPS)
Susac's syndrome
Sympathetic ophthalmia (SO)

T

Takayasu's arteritis
Temporal arteritis/giant cell
  arteritis
Thrombocytopenic purpura
  (TTP)

Thrombotic thrombocytopenic
  purpura (Ttp)
Thyroid eye disease (Ted)
Tolosa-Hunt syndrome (THS)
Transverse myelitis
Type 1 diabetes

U

Ulcerative colitis (UC)
Undifferentiated connective
  tissue disease (UCTD)
Uveitis

V

Vasculitis
Vertigo
Vitiligo
Vogt-Koyanagi-Harada disease

W

Warm autoimmune hemolytic
  anaemia

Further Information

Australian Sleep Health Foundation – sleephealthfoundation.org.au

Sleep Foundation USA – sleepfoundation.org

National Sleep Foundation – thensf.org

Health Direct Australia – healthdirect.gov.au

Australian Institute of Family Studies – aifs.gov.au

Australian Brain Coaching - australianbraincoaching.com.au

Acknowledgments

This book was written on the lands of the Kamilaroi people on the black soil plains of North West New South Wales. I wish to acknowledge and appreciate the people who in the past, present, and future are looking after the land on which we live.

Waking up one day and saying, "I think I'll write a book," sounds easy. Well, having an idea and turning it into a book is not that simple.

It is both challenging and rewarding. I especially want to thank the following people who helped make it happen:

Many thanks to the team at Ultimate World Publishing, who explained the process and nurtured my journey of being a first-time author over the last 3 years, making it less daunting.

Julia Petzl-Berney, for initial proofreading and editing and for being my sounding board; and to Theresa Laas, for design and production of the concise E-book version. Thank you both, for your expertise, support and encouragement.

Elizabeth Tout, for early advice on layout, and for help with the concise E-book version. Your professional advice is very much appreciated.

Cora Besser-Siegmund, Hamburg, for Wing Wave Training, back in 2014, and for developing such a wonderful program of retraining the brain. Astrid Ritter, Cologne, for telling me about Wing Wave all those years ago and for her support since then, and to Barbara Simon and Nicole Lordan, for Wingwave support in Australia.

Jaspreet Singh, for monthly, (or intermittent) spiritual and well-being support over the last 10 years. Your belief in me is very much appreciated and valued.

Thank you also to Graeme Compton, for the photograph on the back cover, and for the illustrations. Not only is he an accomplished photographer, but he is also an awesome artist, painter and illustrator. (Check out his website https://www.artgracom.com/)

To Dr. Grace Higgins, for explaining T-cells and the immune system to me.

Huge thank you to Maree Clark, not only for well-being support over the last few years, also for your wise-words mentoring and being an in-depth Beta-reader and advisor. I am most grateful for your rigorous and thoughtful insight in reading and making suggestions for my manuscript i.e. "What would a reader want to know?". Your mentoring is also majorly appreciated.

To all the many sleep researchers and organisations around the world, working to understand the importance of sleep, and spreading the word on the impact of sleep, or lack of, to society.

To my clients who have improved their sleep and helped spread the word about Brain Coaching. Your belief in the method and following up with your new habits is reaping rewards.

Acknowledgments

To my friends, for their on-going support and encouragement. It means a lot to me. I can't say more than that – you are all amazing.

To my parents, for instilling in me a sense of duty to help others, and for a very strong work ethic. I hope I have inherited at least some of these attributes from them. They will always be remembered.

To my family, husband - Rob, and children - Alex and Anna, for their support and honesty and who haven't minded when I burrowed myself away to write and gnash my teeth about content – you are my reason for being. And special thanks to Rob, for being my biggest fan and for the best morning coffees, best evening cocktails, and for being the best cook. Where would I be without you?!

Offers

S **leep Diary.** Get a better night's sleep with our unique Sleep Diary, developed by Helen. With this Sleep Diary you'll be able to see patterns emerging and identify areas where you can improve both your sleep quantity and quality. Download it for free, via my website.

Speaker Bio – Looking for an engaging guest speaker? Helen is available to facilitate workshops or present at conferences on a variety of topics including: Communication skills; Goal setting; Motivation; Dealing with Difficult people, Dealing with Phobias; as well as Sleep issues. With Helen's expertise and engaging style, your audience is sure to leave feeling inspired and motivated to improve their well-being.

Sleep guide (7-page e-summary). Get the best night's sleep possible with this Guide. This 7-page summary is packed full of tips on what to do and what not to do. Download it for free on my website. With this guide you will be able to identify suggestions that may work for you and get the restful night's sleep that you deserve.

Free 30-minute introductory session. Unlock your full potential and see how Brain Coaching can help you achieve your goals. Sign up for this free offer via the website. After the introduction, you will decide if Brain Coaching is for you. We will then be able to identify areas where you can improve your cognitive abilities and develop new ways of thinking.

Sleep workshops. Looking for a fun and informative way to learn more about quality sleep? We can arrange workshops via video link or in person for interested groups. Contact us to learn more. With our sleep workshops you will pick up lots of information about the Science of Sleep, and tips about negative habits and positive habits that will impact your sleep. You will then have a pathway that you can follow to having restful sleep from now on. These group workshops are ideal for workplace Health, Safety & Wellness training days.

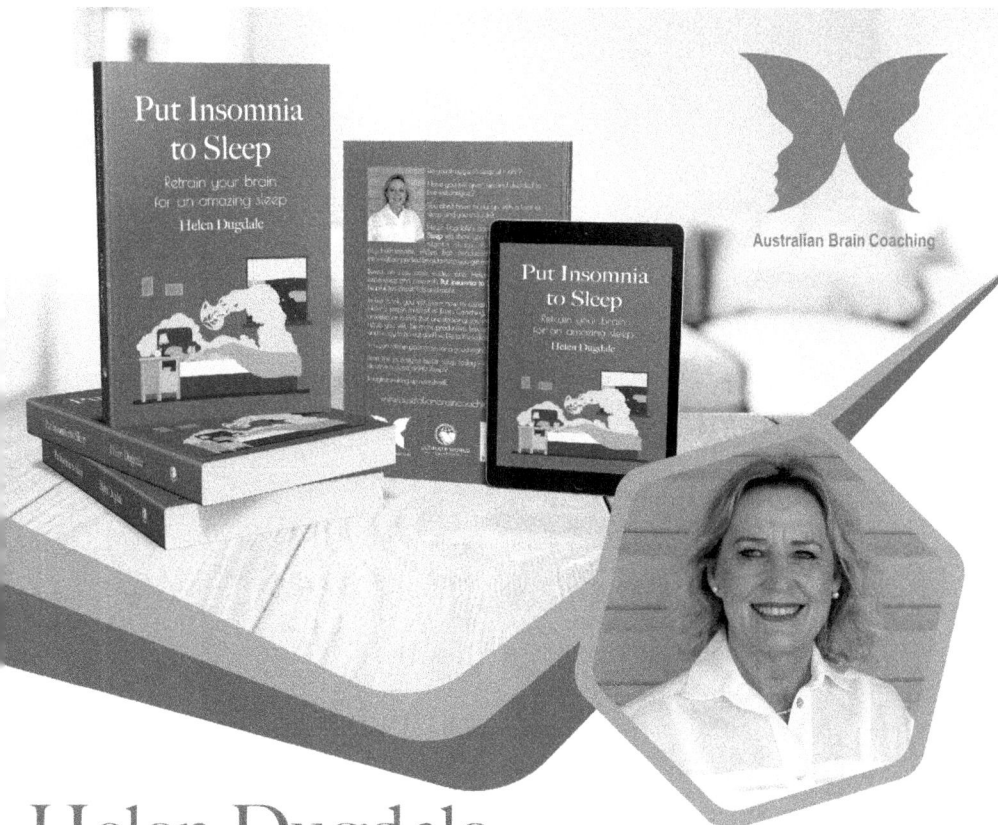

Australian Brain Coaching

Helen Dugdale

Helen Dugdale is the author of Put Insomnia to Sleep. She graduated from the University of New England in 2018 with a Post Graduate Diploma in Psychology and has been running her own business since 2011 delivering personal development programs, sleep workshops and one-on-one Brain Coaching consultations.

Brain coaching helps you to pinpoint and resolve your anxious thinking to lead a more productive and fulfilling life. Helen has been showing clients how it is possible to re-train your brain! While so many people suffer from sleep problems, Helen's clients are having success in overcoming their insomnia.

Just imagine how refreshed and energised you will feel after a great night's sleep. You will be more productive, healthier, and may even live longer. Helen's insights around clean sleeping habits and strategies to overcome insomnia are changing people's quality of life and transforming their relationships with people around them.

Put Insomnia to Sleep

- Where does insomnia come from?
- The scary side-effects of insomnia
- Brain Training to help with insomnia

Bio-Hacking for a Good Nights Sleep

- Let's Get Physical - what's the problem?
- Emotional triggers that prevent good sleep
- Activities that help you sleep

Brain Training for a Healthy & Relaxed Life

- The secret behind your sleep environment
- Identify, Resolve, Re-Program
- Unlocking motivation for success

www.australianbraincoaching.com.au

helen@australianbraincoaching.com.au 0417 064 507

211

References

Intro:

1. Adams, R., Appleton, S., Taylor, A., McEnvoy, D. & Antic, N. (2017b). *Report to the Sleep Health Foundation 2016 Sleep Health Survey of Australian Adults*. (Research Report). University of Adelaide & Adelaide Institute for Sleep Health.

Ch 1.

1. Insomnia. (n.d.) In APA *Dictionary of Psychology*. American Psychological Association. Retrieved November 08, 2022. https://dictionary.apa.org/insomnia

2. Mitler, M. M., Carskadon, M. A., Czeisler, C. A., Dement, W. C., Dinges, D. F, Graeber, R. C. (1988). Catastrophes, sleep, and public policy: consensus report. *Sleep*, 11(1), 100-9. https://doi.org/10.1093/sleep/11.1.100 .

3. Bahrami-Nejad, Z., Zhao, M. L., Tholen, S., Hunerdosse, D., Tkach, K. E., van Schie, S., & Teruel, M. N. (2018). A transcriptional circuit filters oscillating circadian hormonal inputs to regulate fat cell differentiation. *Cell metabolism*, 27(4), 854-868.

4. Calhoun, D. A., Harding, S. M. (2010). Sleep and hypertension. *Chest*, 138(2), 434-43. https://doi.org/10.1378/chest.09-2954

5. Sundelin, T., Lekander, M., Kecklund, G., Van Someren, E. J., Olsson, A., & Axelsson, J. (2013). Cues of fatigue: effects of sleep deprivation on facial appearance. *Sleep*, 36(9), 1355-1360.

6. Oyetakin-White, P., Suggs, A., Koo, B., Matsui, M. S., Yarosh, D., Cooper, K. D., & Baron, E. D. (2015). Does poor sleep quality affect skin ageing? *Clinical and Experimental Dermatology*, 40(1), 17–22. https://doi.org/10.1111/ced.12455

Ch 2.

1. Medic, G., Wille, M., & Hemels, M. E. (2017). Short- and long-term health consequences of sleep disruption. *Nature and science of sleep*, *9*, 151–161. https://doi.org/10.2147/NSS.S134864

2. Alcoholism: Clinical & Experimental Research. (2013, January 22). Reviewing alcohol's effects on normal sleep. *ScienceDaily*. Retrieved January 14, 2023, from www.sciencedaily.com/releases/2013/01/130122162236.htm

3. Wassing, R., Benjamins, J. S., Dekker, K., Moens, S., Spiegelhalder, K., Feige, B., Riemann, D., van der Sluis, S., Van Der Werf, Y. D., Talamini, L. M., Walker, M. P., Schalkwijk, F., & Van Someren, E. J. W. (2016). Slow dissolving of emotional distress contributes to hyperarousal. *Proceedings of the National Academy of Sciences*, *113*(9), 2538–2543. https://doi.org/10.1073/pnas.1522520113

4. Costandi, M. (2018) http://www.wildculture.com/article/cleaning-dirty-brain/1708

5. Paturel, T. (2014). Sleep Well: Could getting more high-quality sleep protect the brain? *Neurology Now*, *10*(1), 34–37. https://doi.org/10.1097/01.NNN.0000444223.41706.4a

6. Daghlas, I., Dashti, H. S., Lane, J., Aragam, K. G., Rutter, M. K., Saxena, R., & Vetter, C. (2019). Sleep duration and myocardial infarction. Journal of the American College of Cardiology, 74(10), 1304–1314., Retrieved November 30, 2020, from https://pubmed.ncbi.nlm.nih.gov/31488267/

7. Shah, N. M., Malhotra, A. M., & Kaltsakas, G. (2020). Sleep disorder in patients with chronic liver disease: a narrative review. *Journal of thoracic disease*, *12*(Suppl 2), S248–S260. https://doi.org/10.21037/jtd-cus-2020-012

8. NIH/National Heart, Lung and Blood Institute. "Poor sleep linked to increased risk of COPD flare-ups." ScienceDaily. ScienceDaily, 6 June 2022. <www.sciencedaily.com/releases/2022/06/220606134411.htm>.

9. Sharma, S., & Kavuru, M. (2010). Sleep and metabolism: an overview. *International journal of endocrinology*, *2010*, 270832. https://doi.org/10.1155/2010/270832

10. Ibarra-Coronado, E. G., Pantaleón-Martínez, A. M., Velazquéz-Moctezuma, J., Prospéro-García, O., Méndez-Díaz, M., Pérez-Tapia, M.,

Pavón, L., & Morales-Montor, J. (2015). The Bidirectional Relationship between Sleep and Immunity against Infections. Journal of immunology research, 2015, 678164. https://www. hindawi.com/journals/jir/2015/678164/.

11. Vandekerckhove, M., & Wang, Y. L. (2017). Emotion, emotion regulation and sleep: An intimate relationship. *AIMS Neuroscience*, *5*(1), 1–17. https://doi.org/10.3934/Neuroscience.2018.1.1

Ch 3.
1. Bonnet, M. H., Arand, D. L. (2019, February 20). Behavioural and pharmacologic therapies for chronic insomnia in adults. *UpToDate.*

2. Scripps Health. (2012, February 27). Higher death risk with sleeping pills. *ScienceDaily.* Retrieved January 14, 2023, from www.sciencedaily.com/releases/2012/02/120227204830.htm

3. Weich, S., Pearce, H. L., Croft, S,. Singh, I., Crome, J., Bashford, J., Frisher, M. (2014) Effect of anxiolytic and hypnotic drug prescriptions on mortality hazards: retrospective cohort study. *BMJ*, *348*(5), g1996-g1996. https://doi.org/10.1136/bmj.g1996

Ch 4.
1. Okamoto-Mizuno, K., & Mizuno, K. (2012). Effects of thermal environment on sleep and circadian rhythm. *Journal of Physiological Anthropology, 31*(1), 14. https://pubmed.ncbi.nlm.nih.gov/22738673/

2. Pape, S. (2017). *The Barefoot Investor: The Only Money Guide You'll Ever Need.* John Wiley & Sons.

3. Choice magazine review. July 2020

Ch 5.
1. Smith, R. P., Easson, C., Lyle, S. M., Kapoor, R., Donnelly, C. P., Davidson, E. J., Parikh, E., Lopez, J. V., & Tartar, J. L. (2019). Gut microbiome diversity is associated with sleep physiology in humans. *PloS one*, *14*(10), e0222394. https://doi.org/10.1371/journal.pone.0222394

2. Snelson, M., de Pasquale, C., Ekinci, E. I., & Coughlan, M. T. (2021). Gut microbiome, prebiotics, intestinal permeability and diabetes complications. *Best practice & research. Clinical endocrinology & metabolism*, *35*(3), 101507. https://doi.org/10.1016/j.beem.2021.101507

3. Quigley, E. M. (2017). Basic definitions and concepts: Organization of the gut microbiome. *Gastroenterology Clinics of North America*, *46*(1), 1-8.

4. Garbarino, S., Lanteri, P., Bragazzi, N. L., Magnavita, N., & Scoditti, E. (2021). Role of sleep deprivation in immune-related disease risk and outcomes. *Communications Biology*, *4*(1), 1304–1304. https://doi.org/10.1038/s42003-021-02825-4

5. Guy-Evans, O. (2021, May 18). Parasympathetic nervous system functions. *Simply Psychology*. www.simplypsychology.org/parasympathetic-nervous-system.html

6. Tsatsis, R. (n.d.). Anxiety Recovery Centre Victoria. Retrieved February 22, 2023, from https://www.arcvic.org.au/34-resources/402-vagus-nerve-exercises

7. Breit, S., Kupferberg, A., Rogler, G., & Hasler, G. (2018). Vagus Nerve as Modulator of the Brain-Gut Axis in Psychiatric and Inflammatory Disorders. *Frontiers in Psychiatry*, *9*, 44–44. https://doi.org/10.3389/fpsyt.2018.00044

8. Kline, C. E. (2014). The bidirectional relationship between exercise and sleep: Implications for exercise adherence and sleep improvement. *American Journal of Lifestyle Medicine*, *8*(6), 375-379. https://doi.org/10.1177/1559827614544437

9. Kline. (2016). Exercise: shifting fluid and sleep apnoea away. *The European Respiratory Journal*, *48*(1), 23–25. https://doi.org/10.1183/13993003.00797-2016

10. Bray, MS., Collica S., Peters, M.E., Tamashiro, K.L. (2020). Exercise Interventions for Mental Health. *Johns Hopkins Psychiatry Guide*. https://www.hopkinsguides.com/hopkins/view/Johns_Hopkins_Psychiatry_Guide/787374/all/Exercise_Interventions_for_Mental_Health

11. Pacecho, D., & Singh, A. (2023, February 8). How can exercise affect sleep? *Sleep Foundation*. *Retrieved* February 22, 2023, from https://www.sleepfoundation.org/physical-activity/exercise-and-sleep

12. Binks, Vincent, G. E., Gupta, C., Irwin, C., & Khalesi, S. (2020). Effects of Diet on Sleep: A Narrative Review. *Nutrients*, *12*(4), 936–. https://doi.org/10.3390/nu12040936

13. Vlahoyiannis, A., Giannaki, C. D., Sakkas, G. K., Aphamis, G., & Andreou, E. (2021). A Systematic Review, Meta-Analysis and Meta-Regression

on the Effects of Carbohydrates on Sleep. *Nutrients*, *13*(4), 1283–. https://doi.org/10.3390/nu13041283

14. Gangwisch, J. E., Hale, L., St-Onge, M. P., Choi, L., LeBlanc, E. S., Malaspina, D., Opler, M. G., Shadyab, A. H., Shikany, J. M., Snetselaar, L., Zaslavsky, O., & Lane, D. (2020). High glycemic index and glycemic load diets as risk factors for insomnia: analyses from the Women's Health Initiative. *The American journal of clinical nutrition*, *111*(2), 429–439. https://doi.org/10.1093/ajcn/nqz275

15. Um, M., Kim, J. Y., Han, J. K., Kim, J., Yang, H., Yoon, M., Kim, J., Kang, S. W., & Cho, S. (2018). Phlorotannin supplement decreases wake after sleep onset in adults with self-reported sleep disturbance: A randomized, controlled, double-blind clinical and polysomnographic study. *Phytotherapy Research*, *32*(4), 698–704. https://doi.org/10.1002/ptr.6019

16. St-Onge, M-P., Mikic, A., & Pietrolungo, C. E. (2016). Effects of diet on sleep quality. *Advances in Nutrition*, *7*(5), 938–949. https://doi.org/10.3945/an.116.012336

17. Lin, H-H., Tsai, P.S., Fang, S.C., & Liu, J.F. (2011). Effect of kiwifruit consumption on sleep quality in adults with sleep problems. *Asia Pacific Journal of Clinical Nutrition*, *20*(2), 169–174. https://doi.org/10.6133/apjcn.2011.20.2.05

18. Bannai, M., & Kawai, N. (2012). New therapeutic strategy for amino acid medicine: Glycine improves the quality of sleep. *Journal of Pharmacological Sciences*, *118*(2), 145–148. https://doi.org/10.1254/jphs.11R04FM

19. Popkin, B.M., D'Anci, K. E., & Rosenberg, I. H. (2010). Water, hydration, and health. *Nutrition Reviews*, *68*(8), 439–458. https://doi.org/10.1111/j.1753-4887.2010.00304.x

20. Strohl, K. P. (2019, February). Merck Manual Professional Version: Obstructive Sleep Apnea. Retrieved August 13, 2020, from https://www.msdmanuals.com/professional/pulmonary-disorders/sleep-apnea/obstructive-sleep-apnea-osa?autoredirectid=20195

21. Appleton, J. (2018). The Gut-Brain Axis: Influence of microbiota on mood and mental health. *Integrative medicine*, *17*(4), 28–32.

22. *Serotonin*. healthdirect. (n.d.). Retrieved February 22, 2023, from https://www.healthdirect.gov.au/serotonin

23. Singh, T., Ahmed, T. H., Mohamed, N., et al. (March 26, 2022) Does Insufficient Sleep Increase the Risk of Developing Insulin Resistance: A Systematic Review. Cureus 14(3): e23501. doi:10.7759/cureus.23501

24. Jenkins, T., Nguyen, J., Polglaze, K., & Bertrand, P. (2016). Influence of tryptophan and serotonin on mood and cognition with a possible role of the gut-brain axis. *Nutrients, 8*(1), 56. https://pubmed.ncbi.nlm.nih.gov/26805875/

25. *Sleep disturbance and menopause.* (n.d.). Retrieved November 14, 2022, from https://www.menopause.org.au/images/stories/infosheets/docs/AMS_Sleep_Disturbance_and_the_Menopause.pdf

26. Information Sheets - Australasian Menopause Society. (n.d.). Retrieved February 22, 2023, from https://www.menopause.org.au/hp/information-sheets

27. Dueren, A. L., Perach, R., Banissy, J. F. M., Bowling, N. C., Gregory, A. M., & Banissy, M. J. (2022). Associations between tactile intimacy and sleep quality in healthy adults: A systematic review. *Journal of Sleep Research*, 31, e13504. https://doi.org/10.1111/jsr.13504

28. Lastella, M., O'Mullan, C., Paterson, J. L., & Reynolds, A. C. (2019). Sex and sleep: Perceptions of sex as a sleep promoting behavior in the general adult population. *Frontiers in Public Health, 7*, 33–33. https://doi.org/10.3389/fpubh.2019.00033

Ch 6.
1. U.S. Department of Health and Human Services. (n.d.). *Sleep science and sleep disorders.* National Heart Lung and Blood Institute. Retrieved February 22, 2023, from https://www.nhlbi.nih.gov/science/sleep-science-and-sleep-disorders

2. Iftikhar, I. H., Kline, C. E., & Youngstedt, S. D. (2014). Effects of exercise training on sleep apnea: a meta-analysis. *Lung, 192*(1), 175–184. https://doi.org/10.1007/s00408-013-9511-3

3. Pacecho, D., & Singh, A. (2022, March 11). *Could your thyroid be causing sleep problems?* Sleep Foundation. Retrieved February 22, 2023, from https://www.sleepfoundation.org/physical-health/thyroid-issues-and-sleep

4. Department of Health & Human Services. (2001, June 15). *Thyroid - hypothyroidism.* Better Health Channel. Retrieved February 22, 2023, from

https://www.betterhealth.vic.gov.au/health/conditionsandtreatments/thyroid-hypothyroidism

5. U.S. Department of Health and Human Services. (n.d.). *Hyperthyroidism (overactive thyroid)*. National Institute of Diabetes and Digestive and Kidney Diseases. Retrieved February 22, 2023, from https://www.niddk.nih.gov/health-information/endocrine-diseases/hyperthyroidism

6. Vadivelu, N., Kai, A. M., Kodumudi, G., Babayan, K., Fontes, M., & Burg, M. M. (2017). Pain and Psychology-A Reciprocal Relationship. *The Ochsner journal*, *17*(2), 173–180.

7. Rampes, S., Ma, K., Divecha, Y. A., Alam, A., & Ma, D. (2019). Postoperative sleep disorders and their potential impacts on surgical outcomes. *Journal of biomedical research*, *34*(4), 271–280. https://doi.org/10.7555/JBR.33.20190054

8. Childs, C. E., Calder, P. C., & Miles, E. A. (2019). Diet and Immune Function. *Nutrients*, *11*(8), 1933. https://doi.org/10.3390/nu11081933

9. Zielinski, M. R., Systrom, D. M., & Rose, N. R. (2019). Fatigue, Sleep, and Autoimmune and Related Disorders. *Frontiers in immunology*, *10*, 1827. https://doi.org/10.3389/fimmu.2019.01827

10. Taylor, D.J., Kelly, K., Kohut, M. L., & Song, K.-S. (2017). Is Insomnia a Risk Factor for Decreased Influenza Vaccine Response? *Behavioral Sleep Medicine*, *15*(4), 270–287. https://doi.org/10.1080/15402002.2015.1126596

11. Besedovsky, L., Lange, T., & Born, J. (2012). Sleep and immune function. *Pflugers Archiv : European journal of physiology*, *463*(1), 121–137. https://doi.org/10.1007/s00424-011-1044-0

12. Krueger, J. M., & Opp, M. R. (2016). Sleep and Microbes. *International review of neurobiology*, *31*, 207–225. https://doi.org/10.1016/bs.irn.2016.07.003

13. *Narcolepsy*. Brain Foundation. (2022, January 18). Retrieved February 22, 2023, from https://brainfoundation.org.au/disorders/narcolepsy/

14. de Oliveira, C.O., Carvalho, L. B., Carlos, K., Conti, C., de Oliveira, M. M., Prado, L. B., & Prado, G. F. (2016). Opioids for restless legs syndrome. *Cochrane Database of Systematic Reviews*, *2016*(6), CD006941–CD006941. https://doi.org/10.1002/14651858.CD006941.pub2

15. Pistorius, F., Geisler, P., Wetter, T. C., & Crönlein, T. (2020). Sleep apnea syndrome comorbid with and without restless legs syndrome: differences

in insomnia specific symptoms. *Sleep & breathing, Schlaf & Atmung, 24(3),* 1167–1172. https://doi.org/10.1007/s11325-020-02063-8

16. Mayo Foundation for Medical Education and Research. (2022, March 1). *Restless legs syndrome.* Mayo Clinic. Retrieved February 22, 2023, from https://www.mayoclinic.org/diseases-conditions/restless-legs-syndrome/diagnosis-treatment/drc-20377174

17. Leung, W., Singh, I., McWilliams, S., Stockler, S., & Ipsiroglu, O. S. (2020). Iron deficiency and sleep - A scoping review. *Sleep medicine reviews, 51,* 101274. https://doi.org/10.1016/j.smrv.2020.101274

18. Otocka-Kmiecik, A., & Król, A. (2020). The role of vitamin C in two distinct physiological states: Physical activity and sleep. *Nutrients, 12*(12), 3908. https://doi.org/10.3390/nu12123908

19. Djokic, G., Vojvodić, P., Korcok, D., Agic, A., Rankovic, A., Djordjevic, V., Vojvodic, A., Vlaskovic-Jovicevic, T., Peric-Hajzler, Z., Matovic, D., Vojvodic, J., Sijan, G., Wollina, U., Tirant, M., Thuong, N. V., Fioranelli, M., & Lotti, T. (2019). The Effects of Magnesium - Melatonin - Vit B Complex Supplementation in Treatment of Insomnia. *Open access Macedonian journal of medical sciences, 7*(18), 3101–3105. https://doi.org/10.3889/oamjms.2019.771

20. *What is Nocturia?* National Association for Continence. (2022, September 27). Retrieved February 22, 2023, from https://nafc.org/nocturia/

21. Irwin, M.R., Carrillo, C., Sadeghi, N., Bjurstrom, M. F., Breen, E. C., & Olmstead, R. (2022). Prevention of Incident and Recurrent Major Depression in Older Adults with Insomnia: A Randomized Clinical Trial. *JAMA Psychiatry (Chicago, Ill.), 79*(1), 33–41. https://doi.org/10.1001/jamapsychiatry.2021.3422

Ch 7.

1. *Sleep and mental health – Harvard health publishing.* Harvard Health. (2021, August 17). Retrieved February 28, 2023, from https://www.health.harvard.edu/newsletter_article/sleep-and-mental-health

2. Nutt, D., Wilson, S., & Paterson, L. (2008). Sleep disorders as core symptoms of depression. *Dialogues in clinical neuroscience, 10*(3), 329–336. https://doi.org/10.31887/DCNS.2008.10.3/dnutt

3. Vandekerckhove, M., & Wang, Y.-L. (2018). Emotion, emotion regulation and sleep: An intimate relationship. *AIMS Neuroscience, 5*(1), 1–22. https://doi.org/10.3934/Neuroscience.2018.1.1

4. Tamm, S., Schwarz, J., Thuné, H., Kecklund, G., Petrovic, P., Åkerstedt, T., Fischer, H., Lekander, M., & Nilsonne, G. (2020). A combined fMRI and EMG study of emotional contagion following partial sleep deprivation in young and older humans. *Scientific reports*, *10*(1), 17944. https://doi.org/10.1038/s41598-020-74489-9

5. Simon, E. B., Oren, N., Sharon, H., Kirschner, A., Goldway, N., Okon-Singer, H., Tauman, R., Deweese, M. M., Keil, A., & Hendler, T. (2015). Losing Neutrality: The Neural Basis of Impaired Emotional Control without Sleep. *The Journal of neuroscience : the official journal of the Society for Neuroscience*, *35*(38), 13194–13205. https://doi.org/10.1523/JNEUROSCI.1314-15.2015

6. Gross, C. R., Kreitzer, M. J., Reilly-Spong, M., Wall, M., Winbush, N. Y., Patterson, R., Mahowald, M., & Cramer-Bornemann, M. (2011). Mindfulness-based stress reduction versus pharmacotherapy for chronic primary insomnia: a randomized controlled clinical trial *Explore*, *7*(2), 76–87. https://doi.org/10.1016/j.explore.2010.12.003

7. Rusch, H. L., Rosario, M., Levison, L. M., Olivera, A., Livingston, W. S., Wu, T., & Gill, J. M. (2019). The effect of mindfulness meditation on sleep quality: a systematic review and meta-analysis of randomized controlled trials. *Annals of the New York Academy of Sciences*, *1445*(1), 5–16. https://doi.org/10.1111/nyas.13996

8. Sharma, M., & Rush, S. E. (2014). Mindfulness-based stress reduction as a stress management intervention for healthy individuals: A systematic review. *Journal of Evidence-Based Complementary & Alternative Medicine, 19*(4), 271–286. https://doi.org/10.1177/2156587214543143

9. Desbordes, G., Negi, L. T., Pace, T. W., Wallace, B. A., Raison, C. L., & Schwartz, E. L. (2012). Effects of mindful-attention and compassion meditation training on amygdala response to emotional stimuli in an ordinary, non-meditative state. *Frontiers in human neuroscience*, *6*, 292. https://doi.org/10.3389/fnhum.2012.00292

10. *Everyday mindfulness with Jon Kabat-Zinn*. Mindful. (2022, October 18). Retrieved February 28, 2023, from https://www.mindful.org/everyday-mindfulness-with-jon-kabat-zinn

11. Luberto, C., Hall, D. L., Park, E. R., Haramati, A., & Cotton, S. (2020). A Perspective on the Similarities and Differences Between Mindfulness and Relaxation. *Global Advances in Health and Medicine, 9*, 2164956120905597–2164956120905597. https://doi.org/10.1177/2164956120905597

12. Davidson, R. J., & Lutz, A. (2008). Buddha's Brain: Neuroplasticity and Meditation. *IEEE signal processing magazine*, *25*(1), 176–174. https://doi.org/10.1109/msp.2008.4431873

13. Franzen, P. L., & Buysse, D. J. (2008). Sleep disturbances and depression: risk relationships for subsequent depression and therapeutic implications. *Dialogues in clinical neuroscience*, *10*(4), 473–481. https://doi.org/10.31887/DCNS.2008.10.4/plfranzen

14. Scott, A. J., Webb, T. L., Martyn-St James, M., Rowse, G., & Weich, S. (2021). Improving sleep quality leads to better mental health: A meta-analysis of randomised controlled trials. *Sleep medicine reviews*, *60*, 101556. https://doi.org/10.1016/j.smrv.2021.101556

Ch 8.
1. Michel, L. C., McCormick, E. M., & Kievit, R. A. (2023). Grey and white matter metrics demonstrate distinct and complementary prediction of differences in cognitive performance in children: Findings from ABCD (N= 11 876). *bioRxiv : the preprint server for biology*, 2023.03.06.529634. https://doi.org/10.1101/2023.03.06.529634)

2. Tarokh, L., Saletin, J. M., & Carskadon, M. A. (2016). Sleep in adolescence: Physiology, cognition and mental health. *Neuroscience and biobehavioral reviews*, *70*, 182–188. https://doi.org/10.1016/j.neubiorev.2016.08.008

3. Taki, Y., Hashizume, H., Thyreau, B., Sassa, Y., Takeuchi, H., Wu, K., Kotozaki, Y., Nouchi, R., Asano, M., Asano, K., Fukuda, H., & Kawashima, R. (2012). Sleep duration during weekdays affects hippocampal gray matter volume in healthy children. *NeuroImage*, *60*(1), 471–475. https://doi.org/10.1016/j.neuroimage.2011.11.072

4. Telzer, E. H., Goldenberg, D., Fuligni, A. J., Lieberman, M. D., & Gálvan, A. (2015). Sleep variability in adolescence is associated with altered brain development. *Developmental cognitive neuroscience*, *14*, 16–22. https://doi.org/10.1016/j.dcn.2015.05.007

5. Kernisan, L. retrieved: https://betterhealthwhileaging.net/

6. *What is Alzheimer's?* Alzheimer's Disease and Dementia. (n.d.). Retrieved February 28, 2023, from https://www.alz.org/alzheimers-dementia/what-is-alzheimers

7. *Alzheimer's study explains how tau pathology affects brain cells.* (2021, July 29). University of Washington Medicine Memory and Brain Wellness Center. https://depts.washington.edu/mbwc/news/article/nuclear-speckles

8. Brzecka, A., Leszek, J., Ashraf, G. M., Ejma, M., Ávila-Rodriguez, M. F., Yarla, N. S., Tarasov, V. V., Chubarev, V. N., Samsonova, A. N., Barreto, G. E., & Aliev, G. (2018). Sleep Disorders Associated with Alzheimer's Disease: A Perspective. *Frontiers in neuroscience*, *12*, 330. https://doi.org/10.3389/fnins.2018.00330

9. Lucey B. (2020). It's complicated: The relationship between sleep and Alzheimer's disease in humans. *Neurobiology of Disease*, *144*, 105031-10531 https://doi.org/10.1016/j.nbd.2020.105031

10. Adams et al. (2017); Sleep problems as a risk factor for chronic conditions. Published November 2021 (https://www.aihw.gov.au/getmedia/7e520067-05f1-4160-a38f-520bac8fc96a/aihw-phe-296.pdf.aspx?inline=true)

Ch 9.
1. Nielsen, H. B., Dyreborg, J., Hansen, Å. M., Hansen, J., Kolstad, H. A., Larsen, A. D., Nabe-Nielsen, K., & Garde, A. H. (2019). Shift work and risk of occupational, transport and leisure-time injury. A register-based case-crossover study of Danish hospital workers. *Safety Science*, *120*, 728–734. https://doi.org/10.1016/j.ssci.2019.07.006

2. Bokenberger, K., Sjölander, A., Dahl Aslan, A. K., Karlsson, I. K., Åkerstedt, T., & Pedersen, N. L. (2018). Shift work and risk of incident dementia: a study of two population-based cohorts. *European journal of epidemiology*, *33*(10), 977–987. https://doi.org/10.1007/s10654-018-0430-8

3. Wickwire, E. M., Geiger-Brown, J., Scharf, S. M., & Drake, C. L. (2017). Shift Work and Shift Work Sleep Disorder: Clinical and Organizational Perspectives. *Chest*, *151*(5), 1156–1172. https://doi.org/10.1016/j.chest.2016.12.007

4. WorkCover NSW. (n.d.) *Shiftwork How to devise an effective roster.* WorkCover Publications. http://www.safework.nsw.gov.au/__data/assets/pdf_file/0014/50063/shiftwork_how_to_devise_effective_roster_0225.pdf

5. Redeker, N. S., Caruso, C. C., Hashmi, S. D., Mullington, J. M., Grandner, M., & Morgenthaler, T. I. (2019). Workplace interventions to promote sleep health and an alert, healthy workforce. *Journal of Clinical Sleep Medicine*, *15*(4), 649–657. https://doi.org/10.5664/jcsm.7734

6. Han, K., Hwang, H., Lim, E., Jung, M., Lee, J., Lim, E., Lee, S., Kim, Y. H., Choi-Kwon, S., & Baek, H. (2021). Scheduled naps improve drowsiness and quality of nursing care among 12-hour shift nurses. *International Journal of Environmental Research and Public Health*, *18*(3), 891. https://doi.org/10.3390/ijerph18030891

7. Cheng, W. J., & Cheng, Y. (2017). Night shift and rotating shift in association with sleep problems, burnout and minor mental disorder in male and female employees. *Occupational and Environmental Medicine*, *74*(7), 483–488. https://doi.org/10.1136/oemed-2016-103898

8. Culpepper, L. (2010). The social and economic burden of shift-work disorder. The Journal of family practice, 59 1 Suppl, S3-S11.

9. Morgenthaler, T.I., Lee-Chiong, T., Alessi, C., Friedman, L., Aurora, R. N., Boehlecke, B., Brown, T., Chesson, A. L., Kapur, V., Maganti, R., Owens, J., Pancer, J., Swick, T. J., & Zak, R. (2007). Practice Parameters for the Clinical Evaluation and Treatment of Circadian Rhythm Sleep Disorders. *Sleep (New York, N.Y.)*, *30*(11), 1445–1459. https://doi.org/10.1093/sleep/30.11.1445

10. Czeisler, C. A., Walsh, J. K., Wesnes, K. A., Arora, S., & Roth, T. (2009). Armodafinil for treatment of excessive sleepiness associated with shift work disorder: a randomized controlled study. *Mayo Clinic Proceedings*, *84*(11), 958–972. https://doi.org/10.1016/S0025-6196(11)60666-6

Ch 10.
1. Bogdan, V.A., Balazsi, R., Lupu, V., (2009). Treating primary insomnia: A comparative study of self-help methods and progressive muscle relaxation. *Journal of Cognitive and Behavioral Psychotherapies*, *9*(1), 67–82. https://www.hopkinsmedicine.org/center-for-music-and-medicine/music-as-medicine.html

Ch 11.
1. Lewis, R. G., Florio, E., Punzo, D., & Borrelli, E. (2021). The brain's reward system in health and disease. *Advances in Experimental Medicine and Biology*, 1344, 57–69. https://doi.org/10.1007/978-3-030-81147-1_4

About the Author

Helen Dugdale has been a science teacher, a trainer, and worked in scientific research management. Her passion for making a difference to people's lives led her to coordinate personal development programs for women, unemployed people, young people, and people in rural areas, to build their skills and confidence. Helen runs her own business delivering workshops, as well as providing one-on-one Brain Coaching consultations. Helen divides her time between regional NSW, Sydney, and Melbourne, seeing clients, as well as spending time with her grandchildren. In her spare time, she enjoys setting challenges for herself. So far, she has climbed Kilimanjaro at age 55, ran her first marathon at age 57 (in London), walked 450km of the French Camino (just before Covid lockdown), graduated from the University of New England with a Post Graduate Diploma in Psychology and is the author of Put Insomnia to Sleep. Helen's next challenge is to go Sky Diving.

Brain-coaching helps you to change your negative ways of thinking to lead a more productive and fulfilling life. Helen is passionate about education and helping people to get the best out of themselves and the people around them. She has qualifications in science; education; training; and psychology.

It is possible to re-train your brain.

www.australianbraincoaching.com.au

Testimonials

Helen Dugdale's book about insomnia is a breath of fresh air. Her no-nonsense practical approach makes the advice and tips presented in the book are straightforward and clear. Printable charts and coloured boxes clearly displaying important information in easy-to-digest dot points place this book ahead of the field.

For readers who are interested in the science behind sleep and the medical side of the problem, the book is packed with well-researched information. Helen Dugdale uses her expertise in this area to create an intricate picture of interlocking systems which all affect our sleep. There is information for people of different ages, for people with medical conditions and for people with lifestyle issues, such as shift work or frequent travel.

Unique to the book is Helen's innovative Brain Coaching approach. Based on the well-documented knowledge that the brain is plastic and can be retrained, Brain Coaching is derived from the WingWave psychological method developed in Germany. In fact, Helen has been specially trained in Europe, to qualify as a WingWave practitioner. Once shown, anyone can apply the simple relaxation techniques which activate both hemispheres of the brain to help them sleep and improve their quality of life.

Julia, Academic, Armidale, NSW

"Imagine what it will feel like to reduce the stress in your life, enjoy the people around you, eliminate the dread of going to bed and getting a full night's sleep. This handy and practical book is for you."

Essie Dempster, Student Counsellor, Adelaide

"Helen has greatly improved my sleep pattern to a restful night with the deep breathing & counting techniques - I now wake feeling calm & refreshed after many years of disturbed & unpleasant thoughts during the night.

I greatly appreciate her kindness & support & highly recommend this sleep technique to all age groups !!!"

George, Farmer, Regional NSW

"This book is an incredible gift for your brain and body. Take it to bed with you tonight! Or the train, bus, park bench - enjoy this resource wherever you are!

Better sleep could be the therapy you need! Helen will guide you to surprising, beautiful results through her thoughtful, evidence-based work.

Sleep - we all do it and we can all benefit from improving! Helen's words will guide the way. Do yourself a favour and absorb this book!"

Kerrie Phipps
Speaker and Leadership Coach, Author of
- Do Talk To Strangers - How to Connect With Anyone,
Anywhere (2014)
- Lifting the Lid on Quiet Achievers - Success Stories of
Regional Entrepreneurs (2010)

"One word to describe Australian Brain Coaching is "WOW"!!! I have never felt better or slept better. Would highly recommend this method to anyone!!! Thank you so much, Helen."

Terri, Northern NSW

"My sleep is so much better since our sessions. I feel so rested in the mornings and energised throughout the day! Helen, your method is definitely helping to improve lives. Thank you so much."

Clare S, Nelson Bay, NSW

"Thank you, Brain Coach – I have gone from 2 hours per night for 30 years, to 7 or 8 hours per night, every night. I can't believe how good I feel!."

Sean, Teacher, North West NSW

"After trying many different therapies, Helen's Brain Coaching method is a breakthrough psychological treatment for me, that can get to the root cause of emotional or performance issues. It is a remarkable, insightful, and an enlightening experience."

Maddison, Port Stephens, NSW